Table of contents

Keto Meal Prep 2020

- **INTRODUCTION** 3
- **THE KETOGENIC DIET AND ITS BENEFITS** 4
  - Benefits 4
  - Maintaining the Ketogenic Diet 5
  - Why Keto? 5
  - What About Diabetics? 6
  - Living with Ratios 7
  - Nutrients that are Needed 8
  - Getting Ready 8
- **KETOSIS AND ITS EFFECTS** 9
  - Getting into Ketosis 9
  - Reaching Optimal Levels of Ketosis 10
  - Ketosis and Ketoacidosis 11
  - Brain Fuel 11
  - Measuring Ketosis 12
- **KETO KITCHEN STAPLES** 15
  - Clean out the Pantry 15
  - Go Shopping 19
  - Getting the Kitchen Ready 26
- **MEAL PREP** 28
  - Begin Simple 28
  - Meal Prep Ideas 28
  - Storage 29
  - Mistakes to Avoid 32
- **MEAL PREP FOR BEGINNERS** 34
  - WEEK ONE Shopping List 35
  - WEEK ONE Prep 38
  - WEEK TWO Shopping List 45
  - WEEK TWO Prep 47
- **MEAL PREP FOR PERFORMANCE** 54
  - WEEK ONE Shopping List 55
  - WEEK ONE Prep 57
  - WEEK TWO Shopping List 64
  - WEEK TWO Prep 66
- **MEAL PREP FOR MAINTENANCE** 70
  - WEEK ONE Shopping List 71
  - WEEK ONE Prep 74
  - WEEK TWO Shopping List 79
  - WEEK TWO Prep 81
- **BREAKFAST** 86
- **MAIN DISHES** 109

SPECIALTY, DESSERT, AND SNACKS	157
CONCLUSION	182
DESCRIPTION	183

30-DAY KETOGENIC MEAL PLAN

INTRODUCTION	186
THE BASICS	187
THE PRINCIPLES	187
GUIDELINES	188
CREATING A MEAL PLAN	190
STICKING WITH THE DIET	192
30-DAY MEAL PLAN	193
BREAKFAST	197
AVOCADO MILKSHAKE	197
GRANOLA	197
PEANUT BUTTER SMOOTHIE	198
CREAM CHEESE PANCAKES	199
KETO COFFEE	199
LEMON SMOOTHIE	200
BREAKFAST BAKE	200
GREEN SMOOTHIE	201
AVOCADO AND EGGS	202
BERRY SHAKE	203
BREAKFAST CRÈME	203
CHIA BERRY SMOOTHIE BOWL	204
GOAT CHEESE OMELET	204
BLUEBERRY MUFFIN	205
CINNAMON CHIA PUDDING	206
CACAO CHIA SHAKE	207
EVERYTHING BAGEL	207
EGG MUFFIN CUP	208
LATKES	209
MUSHROOM FRITTATA	210
ARTICHOKE AND BACON OMELET	211
CAPRESE OMELET	212
LUNCH	213
CHICKEN WRAPS	213
GRILLED SALMON AND ASPARAGUS	213
CHICKEN BACON BURGER	214
BOLOGNESE ZOODLES	215
ZESTY TILAPIA	216
AVOCADO PESTO ZOODLES	217
ROASTED CHICKEN WITH VEGGIES	218
SHRIMP SCAMPI WITH ZOODLES	219
TACO ROLLS	220
FAJITA BOWL	221
PORTOBELLO PIZZA	222
CARBONARA	223
PIZZA	224
THAI ZOODLES	225

    Ricotta and Spinach Gnocchi 226

DINNER 228

    Turkey Meatloaf 228
    Haddock 229
    Zucchini Gratin 229
    Cauliflower Mac and Cheese 230
    Lettuce Wrap Cheeseburger 231
    Pork Loin with Mustard Sauce 232
    Lamb with Sun-Dried Tomatoes 233
    Thai Lettuce Wrap 234
    Cheeseburger 235
    Tri-Tip 236
    Sausage Casserole 236
    Sausage Crust Pizza 237
    Garlic Parmesan Salmon 238
    Coconut Lime Skirt Steak 239
    Creamy Butter Chicken 240
    Buffalo Chicken 241
    Sausage and Veggies 242
    Stuffed Peppers 243
    Crispy Wings 244
    Pulled Pork 245
    Dijon Chicken with Vegetables 246
    Indian-Style Chicken 247
    Mexican Meatloaf 248
    Chicken Enchiladas 249
    Halibut Butter Sauce 250
    Lamb Chops with Tapenade 251
    Sirloin and Butter 252
    Noodles with Beef Stroganoff Meatballs 254
    Chicken Cordon Bleu Casserole 255
    Turkey Mushroom Bake 256
    Turkey Pot Pie 257
    Buttered Duck 258
    Cheesy Salmon 259
    Herbed Scallops 260
    Buttery Lemon Chicken 261
    Stuffed Chicken Breast 262
    Turkey Rissoles 263
    Stuffed Pork Chops 264
    Rosemary Garlic Rack of Lamb 264
    Garlic Short Ribs 265
    Bacon Wrapped Steaks 266
    Italian Burgers 267
    Saffron Shrimp 268
    Pesto Chicken Casserole 269
    Meat Pie 270

SOUPS 272

    Cauliflower Soup 272
    Thai Chicken Soup 273
    Bacon Cheeseburger Soup 274
    Cheesy Broccoli Soup 275
    Beef Stew 275
    Chicken Soup 276

Easy Chicken Chili	277
Turkey and Leek Soup	278
Turkey Chili	279
Turkey Stew	280
Coconut Chicken Soup	281
Mexican Turkey Soup	282
Sun-Dried Tomato and Chicken Stew	282
Cream of Tomato and Thyme Soup	283
Gazpacho	284
Coconut and Shrimp Curry Soup	285
Green Minestrone Soup	286
Shrimp Stew	287
Sausage Beer Soup	288
Wild Mushroom and Thyme Soup	289
Reuben Soup	290

SALADS ... 291

Taco Salad	291
Crab Salad Avocado	292
Tuna Salad	292
BLT Salad	293
Salmon Salad	294
Feta Salad	295
Turkey and Avocado Salad	295
Caesar Salad	296
Brussels Sprouts Salad	297
Avocado Salad	298
Tuna Salad	299
Turkey Salad	300
Steak Salad	301
Tuna Caprese Salad	302
Asian Beef Salad	303
Bacon and Blue Cheese Salad	304
Prawn Salad	305
Garlicky Chicken Salad	306
Strawberry Spinach Salad	307
Warm Artichoke Salad	308
Spinach Bacon Salad	309
Crab Meat Salad	310

TREATS ... 311

Cinnamon Smoothie	311
Blueberry Smoothie	311
Vanilla Ice Cream	312
Brownies	313
Pecan Peanut Butter Bars	313
Peanut Butter Cookie	314
Strawberry Butter	315
Peanut Butter Mousse	315
Peanut Butter Cups	316
Mound Bars	317
Peppermint Mocha Drops	317
Mocha Bonbons	318
Herb Crusted Goat Cheese	319
Coconut Chips	319
Cashew Bars	320

- Pizza Chips 321
- Coconut Candy 322
- Chocolate Mint Fat Bombs 322
- Mini Strawberry Cheesecakes 323
- Avocado Crunch Bombs 323
- Pumpkin Mug Cake 324

SNACKS AND SIDES 326
- Bacon Deviled Eggs 326
- Parmesan Chips 326
- Kale Chips 327
- Bacon Fat Bombs 328
- Golden Rosti 328
- Broccoli Cheddar Tots 329
- Pecorino Mushroom Burgers 330
- Roasted String Beans 332
- Fries and Aioli 332
- Garlic Mashed Celeriac 333
- Spicy Deviled Eggs 334
- Avocado Crostini 335
- Low-Carb Cheddar Bay Biscuits 336
- Spinach and Cheese Balls 337
- Stuffed Piquillo Peppers 338
- Coconut Ginger Macaroons 339
- Chicken Fritters with Dip 340
- Amaretti Biscuits 341
- Pesto Parmesan Dip 342
- Bacon Dip 342
- Cheddar Chips 343
- Nachos 344
- Queso 345
- Parmesan Crackers 345
- Asparagus and Walnuts 346
- Garlicky Green Beans 346
- Creamed Spinach 347
- Zucchini Crisps 348
- Mashed Cheesy Cauliflower 349
- Mushroom and Camembert 349
- Zucchini Noodles with Pesto 350
- Bacon and Blue Cheese Zoodles 351

CONCLUSION 352
DESCRIPTION 353

Keto Meal Prep 2020

The Complete Guide to Keto Meal Prep for Beginners: Burn Fat, Save Money, Save Time, and Live Your Best Life

Tyler MacDonald

© Copyright 2020 by Tyler MacDonald - All rights reserved.

This book is provided with the sole purpose of providing relevant information on a specific topic for which every reasonable effort has been made to ensure that it is both accurate and reasonable. Nevertheless, by purchasing this book you consent to the fact that the author, as well as the publisher, are in no way experts on the topics contained herein, regardless of any claims as such that may be made within. As such, any suggestions or recommendations that are made within are done so purely for entertainment value. It is recommended that you always consult a professional prior to undertaking any of the advice or techniques discussed within.

This is a legally binding declaration that is considered both valid and fair by both the Committee of Publishers Association and the American Bar Association and should be considered as legally binding within the United States.

The reproduction, transmission, and duplication of any of the content found herein, including any specific or extended information will be done as an illegal act regardless of the end form the information ultimately takes. This includes copied versions of the work physical, digital, and audio unless an expressed consent of the Publisher is provided beforehand. Any additional rights reserved.

Furthermore, the information that can be found within the pages described forthwith shall be considered both accurate and truthful when it comes to the recounting of facts. As such, any use, correct or incorrect, of the provided information will render the Publisher free of responsibility as to the actions taken outside of their direct purview. Regardless, there are zero scenarios where the original author or the Publisher can be deemed liable in any fashion for any damages or hardships that may result from any of the information discussed herein.

Additionally, the information in the following pages is intended only for informational purposes and should thus be thought of as universal. As befitting its nature, it is presented without assurance regarding its prolonged validity or interim quality. Trademarks that are mentioned are done without written consent and can in no way be considered an endorsement from the trademark holder.

Introduction

Finding time to prepare healthy meals at home can be a pain, right? You work all day long. You may have children to take care of. You could even be trying to take college courses. With life hitting you from everywhere, when are you supposed to have time to cook? Maybe you have the time to cook, but you want to save money and time so that you can do things with your family or hit the gym.

Chances are that you have a lot that you want to accomplish while also getting healthier. A ketogenic diet is a great option for getting healthy, but it can seem overwhelming at first. There are a lot of people who are in your position. The great news is that learning keto meal prepping will solve your problems.

Throughout this book, you learn about the ketogenic diet as well as meal prep. You will learn exactly what it means to be keto, and how you will lose weight, get healthy, and improve your life with the help of this low-carb high-fat. The list of benefits associated with the ketogenic diet is nearly endless.

The main reason people fail when they first start out on a ketogenic diet is that they don't have easy access to keto-friendly meals. This is especially true for the busy person. They end up not having enough time to make their meals. When you start using meal prepping, it will make this a hundred times easier. For those who have never heard of or tried meal prepping, a simple explanation is that you make all of your meals in advance. Meal prep is essentially homemade TV dinners.

Meal prepping has gained in popularity and it is only going to continue to grow. Meal prepping gives you more control over what you consume and it guarantees you a healthy meal that is just a freezer away. The aim of keto meal prepping is to help make the ketogenic diet easier so that you won't be so quick to turn to non- keto, processed, and packaged foods. This is extremely simple to execute, and you will quickly see the benefits in as little as a week.

The book has three two-week meal prep plans for the beginner, performance minded, and for maintenance. Besides that, there will be several other recipes to follow the meal prep plans. You will also find nutrition information so that you no longer need to worry about figuring it out on your own.

Thank you for choosing *Keto Meal Prep 2020*. Now, if you are ready to get started and feel amazing, let's continue.

The Ketogenic Diet and Its Benefits

Why is everyone so crazy about the keto diet? Well, this low carb diet focuses on you consuming lots of healthy fats while lowering your intake of carbs. You get your energy from consuming only 75 percent fats, 20 percent protein, and 5 percent carbs. This means you are only allowed to eat 20 to 50 grams of carbs each day.

This diet was named for the metabolic process called ketosis, where the body changes its fuel source from carbs to fat that has been stored in the body. The goal of this diet is forcing the body into ketosis which causes your liver to begin producing ketones that will run your body. You aren't starving yourself; you are just keeping carbs away from the body. This could cause improved focus, fast weight loss, better physical health, and improved mental clarity.

The ketogenic diet is a bit like the Atkins diet or any other low carb diets. Once you change the body's fuel source, the body's metabolism will change, and this makes you feel more energized.

Benefits

The ketogenic diet does offer many benefits. Here are a few of the big ones:

- ***Increased Muscle Mass:*** This diet is great if you are looking to increase your muscle mass because you are eating more protein.

- ***Anti-Aging:*** Your skin and body will feel and look younger when you follow this diet.

- ***Decreased Inflammation:*** This diet produces ketone bodies which the body burns better than carbs and, in turn, creates fewer free radicals and less oxidation that damages cell membranes and thus reduces inflammation.

- ***Better Skin:*** Many people have noticed this diet helps soften their skin and can clear up acne.

- ***Increases Energy:*** The keto diet improves mitochondrial function by producing less free radicals.

- ***Improves Brain Function:*** Since the brain runs better off ketones, this diet can help with problems focusing and brain fog.

- ***Reduces the Risk of Many Diseases:*** If you have any of the following conditions, this diet could help improve them:

- High Blood Pressure
- Fatty Liver Disease
- Migraines
- Cancer
- Heart Disease
- Obesity
- Parkinson's Disease
- Chronic Inflammation
- Alzheimer's Disease
- Type 1 Diabetes
- Type 2 Diabetes
- Epilepsy

- ***Quick Weight Loss:*** When you begin the keto diet, you could lose up to ten pounds in your first week. This loss will mainly be excess water weight. After this quick reduction in weight, you could lose up to two pounds per week from there.

Maintaining the Ketogenic Diet

This diet encourages you to eat fresh foods such as healthy oils and fats, vegetables, fish, and meats. You will be reducing all chemically-treated and processed foods. You can do this diet for a long time and even enjoy it. This is essential if you want to lose weight and help with the above conditions. What isn't to love about a diet that lets you eat eggs and bacon for breakfast?

Every study that has been done shows this diet can help people feel fuller longer, have more energy through the day and lose weight. Feeling fuller longer and having more energy comes from the biggest part of your daily calories coming from fats that are digested slower and denser in calories. Because of this, most people who follow this diet will eat fewer calories since they feel fuller longer and don't have cravings.

Why Keto?

Once you begin eating a ketogenic diet, your body will get better at burning fats for fuel. This is wonderful for many reasons. The main reason is that fats have more calories than carbs and this keeps you from eating so much food. Your body easily burns all the fat that has been stored which is what you want to get rid of. This, in turn, results in losing more weight. Burning fat for fuel gives you constant energy and won't cause spikes in your blood glucose. You won't be experiencing the lows and highs you get when eating huge amounts of carbs.

Having constant energy level during your day means you will get more done and won't feel as tired.

Along with these benefits, following a keto diet can also help with:

- Improve brain function
- Improves good or HDL levels of cholesterol
- Reduces bad or LDL levels of cholesterol
- Reduces blood pressure
- Reduces triglyceride levels
- Reduces insulin resistance and blood sugar
- Results in losing more body fat.

What About Diabetics?

If you have been diagnosed with diabetes, you can still do a low carb diet. For anyone who has type 2 diabetes, it could start reversing the condition and for people who have type 1 diabetes, it could improve the way your body controls blood sugar.

Always talk with your doctor before starting a low carb diet, especially if you have type 1 diabetes. If you take medicines to help control your insulin levels, you might have to decrease your dose. Your physician might suggest you begin this diet under their supervision so they can check your blood glucose levels and change up your dose of insulin if needed. If you are type 1 diabetic, you need to eat over 50 grams of carbs each day to keep you from going into ketoacidosis.

Ketoacidosis is a metabolic state that becomes toxic when your body can't regulate its production of ketones. This causes a large accumulation of keto acids that causes the blood's pH to decrease drastically and makes the blood acidic. The main causes of ketoacidosis are extreme starvation, prolonged alcoholism, and
type 1 diabetes. This could result in starvation ketoacidosis, alcoholic ketoacidosis, and diabetic ketoacidosis. Ketoacidosis usually doesn't happen for any reason other than being a type 1 diabetic.

Living with Ratios

The keto diet was built on ratios just like the Food Pyramid. It is extremely important to consume the correct balance of macronutrients so your body gets the energy that is needed so you aren't missing any essential protein or fat.

Foods are made of macronutrients. These include carbohydrates, protein, and fats. Every macronutrient gives you a specific amount of energy for every gram that is eaten.

- Carbs will give you around four calories per gram.
- Protein gives you around four calories per gram.
- Fats give you about nine calories per gram.

With this diet, the calories you should get from fats need to be about 65 to 75 percent. The calories from protein need to be around 20 to 25 percents and the last five percent comes from carbs.

The number of calories you consume all depends on a few different factors:

- Do you want to gain muscle?
- Do you want to maintain the muscles you have?
- Do you want to lose weight?
- The types of workout you do: cardio, weight lifting, or both
- The number of hours you do the above each week.
- Your daily activity level: are you a pro athlete, wait tables, sit behind a desk.
- Your current body weight (lean): the body fat subtracted from the total weight.

You can find a calculator online that will give you your daily macro levels. You can find one by doing a quick search for "keto calculator". These will allow you to quickly and easily put in your numbers and get an estimate for your specific caloric needs.

A great thing about this diet is it isn't important to track every number to reach your goal. If you would like to track it that way, it is a good way to increase your progress. By keeping track, you will get a reminder every day to stay on course.

Nutrients that are Needed

You absolutely have to drink a lot of water when you start the keto diet. You might even realize you are going to the bathroom more often, and this is perfectly normal because your body is getting rid of all your water weight.

This occurs since you have cut out many processed foods and have begun consuming more whole foods. Processed foods are loaded with sodium and when you change up your diet suddenly, it causes a quick drop in your sodium intake.

When you reduce your carb intake, it lowers your insulin levels. This sends a message to your kidneys to get rid of excess sodium. Because the body is getting rid of stored sodium, and by reducing the amount of sodium you are consuming, your body starts getting rid of a lot of water and your body might become low on electrolytes and sodium.

Once this happens, you might have symptoms like nausea, irritability, runny nose, coughing, headaches, and fatigue. This is commonly called the "keto flu". It is important that you understand this isn't the actual influenza virus. This is called the "keto flu" because of the similar symptoms to the actual flu it isn't a real virus or contagious.

Most people who experience these symptoms think this diet is what made them sick and start eating carbs again. This "flu phase" means your body is having withdrawals from processed foods, carbs, and sugar. It is learning to use fat as fuel. The "keto flu" only last a couple of days while your body gets adjusted. You can lessen these symptoms by adding more electrolytes and sodium into your diet.

Getting Ready

Now that you have the information behind the science and benefits of the ketogenic diet, you are ready to start. In the remaining chapters, you are going to get all the information you will need to succeed with this diet, including recipes, meal plans, what foods to stay away from, and what foods to buy.

Ketosis and Its Effects

When you eat a high carb diet, your body is in glycolysis, which is a metabolic state. This means that the majority of the energy your body expends comes from the glucose in your blood. When you are in this state, and after you have eaten, your blood glucose spikes and creates high levels of insulin. This causes your body to store fat. This, in turn, keeps your body from releasing the fat it has stored in its tissues.

Ketosis is a natural state your body enters when it gets fueled by fat. This can happen when you fast or are following a strict low carb diet.

There are many benefits to being in ketosis like weight loss, performance, and health. These can come with some side effects. For people who have type 1 diabetes or other diseases, excessive ketosis can become dangerous.

When you are in ketosis, your body will produce ketones. These are small fuel molecules that the body uses as fuel when the body's glucose supplies are short.
Your fat reserves will continuously be released and then consumed. Your liver will begin converting fat into ketones that get released into the bloodstream. Your body will use these just like glucose. The brain can be fueled by ketones, too.

Getting into Ketosis

There are two ways for the body to reach ketosis: following a ketogenic diet or fasting. With either one of these circumstances, when the body's glucose gets depleted, the body switches its fuel source to fat. Insulin, which is a hormone that stores fat, when it becomes low and your body is burning fat, its ability to burn fat will increase. What this means is that your body will have better access to your fat stores and will be able to get rid of them.

You can consider yourself in ketosis when your body produces enough ketones to make a significant level in the blood, usually more than .5 millimeters. The fastest way for this to happen is by fasting, but you can't fast forever.

This is why most people begin a ketogenic diet since you can eat this diet for an indefinite amount of time.

The goal of this diet is to keep you in ketosis at all times. If you are just beginning this diet, to get your body into ketosis could take anywhere from one to two months.

When your body has gotten into ketosis, the glucose your body has stored in your liver and muscles will decrease, your energy levels will be higher, your muscle endurance will increase, and you will have less water weight. If you knock
yourself out of ketosis due to eating too many carbs, you can return to ketosis

faster than before. When your body becomes adapted to the diet, you can increase your carb intake to 50 grams of carbohydrates each day and still stay in ketosis.

Reaching Optimal Levels of Ketosis

This is the point everyone who does this diet wants to reach. Once you have reached optimal ketosis, your body burns fat at the fastest speed it can. In order to get to this level, you have to follow this diet as stated in this book. There aren't any tricks that will help you reach this level but there are certain things you can do.

Here are the various levels of ketones you could have:

- Under 0.5 means you aren't in ketosis.
- Between 0.5 and 1.5 is a light level of ketosis. In this range, you will lose weight but it isn't going to be optimal.
- About 1.5 to 3 is considered optimal and is best for maximum weight loss.
- Levels over 3 are unnecessary. High levels won't help you in any way. It might harm you since it might mean you are not eating enough food.

There are many people who think that they are following a strict diet but are surprised when they measure their ketone levels. When they measure them, the ketone levels measure about 0.2 or 0.5 which is nowhere near the sweet spot.

The trick to getting over this plateau is you have to steer clear of all the obvious sources of carbs but make sure your intake of protein doesn't go higher than your intake of fats. It has been said that protein won't change your glucose levels as carbs will, but if you eat too many, especially if you consume more protein than fat, it is going to affect your glucose levels. This is going to compromise your optimal ketosis.

The secret to working around this problem is to increase your fat intake. This can easily be done by adding a large dollop of herbed butter to the top of your steak. This can keep you from eating too much or eating a second helping.

You could also start your day with a c of keto coffee to help you not feel hungry before lunch and help you not eat as much protein. You'll find the recipe later on in the book.

The more fat you consume, the fuller you are going to feel. This makes sure you don't eat too much protein, and you are going to eat fewer carbs. This will help you reach optimal ketosis.

Ketosis and Ketoacidosis

There are so many misconceptions about ketosis. The biggest one is confusing it with ketoacidosis. This is a dangerous but rare condition that usually only happens to people who have type 1 diabetes. There are some health care professionals that mix these two up. The main reason might be because their names are similar and there isn't a lot of information on the differences between the two.

Ketosis, as stated above, is a normal state that the body can control. Ketoacidosis is where the body malfunctions because it has created an excessive and unregulated amount of ketones. This can cause things such as vomiting, stomach pain, and nausea. This is then followed by confusion and possibly a coma. This requires urgent medical treatment that might even become fatal.

Ketoacidosis occurs when ketones reach a level of 10 millimolar or more. People that follow a keto diet usually only reach a level of three millimolar or less. There are many people who struggle to reach 0.5. Long-term fasting, which means you haven't consumed food for over one week, could bring that number up to six.

If you have a pancreas that functions properly and produces insulin correctly, mean you don't have type 1 diabetes, it is going to be extremely hard for you to reach ketoacidosis even if you tried. The reason this won't happen is that your body releases insulin when your body produces too many ketones, and this shuts down ketone production. Since type 1 diabetes prevents insulin production, their bodies can't regulate overactive ketones.

Brain Fuel

Many people think you need to eat carbs to have fuel for your brain. Our brains will happily burn carbs when you eat them, but when carbs become unavailable, it will happily eat ketones.

This is needed for basic survival because our bodies can only store carbs for a couple of days. The brain might shut down after a few days without food.
Alternatively, it needs to convert muscle protein quickly into glucose, which isn't efficient just to keep working. This means we might waste away very fast. If this was the way our bodies actually worked, then humans would not have been able to survive before food became available to us 24 hours a day and seven days a week.

Our bodies have evolved to work a lot smarter than that. Normally, our bodies will store fat that will last so we can survive several weeks without any food.
Ketosis is what happens to make sure our brains can run on these fat stores.

Measuring Ketosis

When you begin the keto diet, you need to know when you are in ketosis. This will create a big boost in your confidence. Testing lets you know whether or not you are following the diet correctly.

There are a few ways to help you figure out whether or not you have reached ketosis. The first way to measure ketones is by testing your blood. This means you have to buy a meter and requires you to prick your finger.

There are a few reasonably priced gadgets out there that can help you with this and it only takes a few seconds to figure out what your blood ketone level is.
Many people won't go to this extreme, but it is the most accurate and effective.

You need to measure your blood ketones first thing every morning on a fasted stomach. You can compare them with levels that were listed earlier in this chapter to see if you are or aren't in ketosis.

These meters will measure the amount of BHB you have in your blood. This is the main ketone that is present in the blood when you are in ketosis. The downside of this method is having to prick your finger to get blood.

Finding a kit will cost about $30 to $40, with another $5 for each test strip. This is why most people who choose this test, only performs a test each week or every other week.

If your budget won't allow you to purchase a blood ketone meter, there are other options that will help you figure out whether or not you have reached ketosis.

1. Insomnia

A huge issue for many keto followers is having insomnia, especially when they are just beginning this diet. When a person reduces their carb intake drastically, it could cause sleeping problems. As with everything else, this too shall pass.

2. Short-term fatigue

When your body is making the initial switch into ketosis, it could cause weakness and fatigue, and this makes it hard for many people to stick with it. This is a normal side effect but one that lets you know you are reaching ketosis.

This crappy feeling might last for one week up to one month before you reach full ketosis. In order to reduce this feeling, you could take an electrolyte supplement or add more salt into your diet.

3. Digestive issues

Because of all the changes in the foods you are eating, you may end up experiencing some constipation or diarrhea when just starting out. This lets you know that you are reaching ketosis. Once this transition period is over, these issues should go away.

4. Short-term performance decrease

Just like number two above, fatigue could cause a decrease in your exercise performance. This is because of the reduction in the glycogen stores that were in your muscles that gave you the fuel you needed to do high-intensity exercises.
After a week or two, your performance levels should return to normal.

5. Appetite suppression

Many people report that their hunger decreases when they follow a ketogenic diet. The reason behind this is still being researched. It is believed that this reduction in hunger is caused by the increase in protein and vegetable consumption, along with the changes in your hunger hormones. These ketones might affect the way your brain reacts to hunger.

6. Better focus and energy

Many people sometimes report feeling tired, sick, or having brain fog when they begin a keto diet. This is called the keto flu, but people who follow this for a long time reports increased focus and better energy. Your body needs time to adapt to any new diet. When you hit ketosis, your brain begins burning ketones for energy, and this might take a week or two for it to begin happening.

Ketones are a powerful fuel source for the brain as opposed to carbs. This means it will improve your mental clarity and brain function.

7. Ketones in your breath and urine

If you don't like the thoughts of pricking your finger, you can measure blood ketones by using a breath analyzer. This monitors for acetone, which is one of the three ketones that are present in the blood when you have reached ketosis. The other two are beta-hydroxybutyrate and acetoacetate.

This lets you know when your ketone levels are in ketosis since acetone only leaves your body when you reach ketosis. Breath analyzers are fairly accurate but not as accurate as the blood monitor.

Another way to check for ketosis is by checking for ketones in your urine daily using special strips. These are cheap and quick to use to see where your ketone levels are each day. These aren't very reliable.

8. Bad breath

This doesn't sound appealing at all but many people have said they have bad breath when they hit ketosis. This is a normal side effect. Some people have said that their breath tastes fruitier.

The reason behind this is the elevated ketone levels. The main culprit is acetone that our bodies will excrete through our breath and urine. You might not like the thoughts of having bad breath, but it's a great way to know you are in ketosis.

Many people will brush their teeth many times throughout the day or chew sugar- free gum.

9. *Weight loss*

This is the most obvious way to know that you are in ketosis. When you are just beginning a keto diet, you are going to have a quick drop in weight, but this is normally water weight. Once you have another drop in weight, this will be your fat stores being used. This is another way you know you are in ketosis.

There are many different signs and symptoms that help you know when you are in ketosis, and if you are following the diet correctly. Basically, if you follow the rules for a keto diet and you stay consistent, your body will be in some form of ketosis.

If you want to know for certain whether or not you are in ketosis, the best way to do this is by using a blood ketone monitor.

If you are following this diet for a long time, you don't have to constantly check your ketone levels. After a few weeks, you will know if you are eating right and it will be easy to remain in ketosis.

Keto Kitchen Staples

Now that you know the science behind this diet and the reasons it works, you are going to learn how to start it and maximize your success. Here is an easy guide for you to use when starting this diet. You can even look back at this any time in your journey for guidance and support.

Clean out the Pantry

You've heard the old saying: "Out with the old, in with the new". Keeping unhealthy, tempting foods inside your house is the largest factor of failing when you begin any diet. If you want to succeed, you have to minimize all triggers in order to maximize success. If you don't have the iron-will of DeWayne Johnson, you shouldn't keep foods such as desserts, bread, or other unfriendly snacks.

If you live with others, make sure you talk with and warn them about your new lifestyle changes. If they need to keep some items, find someplace where they can be kept out of sight. This will help everyone who shares your home to understand that you are serious about your new lifestyle. This will lead to a better experience for everyone involved.

Below is a list of foods you need to get rid of and why:

Grains and starches: These foods are very high in carbohydrates. Just a small serving could kick you out of ketosis. You need to eliminate the following:

- Crackers
- Cookies
- Pizza
- Cornstarch
- Beer
- Cornmeal
- Whole Rye
- Brown rice
- Cereals
- Cakes
- Sugar

- Quinoa
- Barley
- Corn
- Wheat
- Pasta
- Rice

Sugary drinks and foods: Sugars have to be avoided at all costs when following the keto diet. Get rid of the following:

- Any product labeled as "low fat"
- Any foods that are processed
- Chocolate
- Sports drinks
- Candy
- Ice cream
- Cakes
- Store-bought smoothies
- Fruit juices
- Maple syrup
- Barley malt syrup
- Dark brown sugar
- Agave nectar
- Molasses
- Sodas
- Light brown sugar

Fruits: Eliminate all fruits that are high in carbs. Dried fruits contain as much sugar as normal fruit but are more concentrated. This makes it easy to eat lots of sugar in a small serving. One c of raisins has more than 100 grams of carbs while a c of grapes only has 15 grams. Get rid of the following:

- Bananas
- Dates
- Grapes
- Mangos
- Apples
- All dried fruits

Legumes and beans: Legumes and beans have moderate amounts of carbs that can damage your keto efforts. Get rid of the following. One c of beans contains three times the amounts of carbs you should eat in one day. Get rid of the following:

- Edamame
- Navy beans
- Lentils
- Mung beans
- Pinto beans
- Peas
- Black beans
- Kidney beans
- Great northern beans

Processed polyunsaturated oils and fats: Eliminate most seed oil and all oils that say "vegetable". Basically, anything labeled as "partially hydrogenated" or "hydrogenated".

- Vegetable oils
- Margarine

- Cottonseed oil
- Canola oil
- Sunflower oil
- Safflower oil
- Soybean oil
- Hydrogenated oil

Root vegetables: These vegetables contain higher amounts of carbs than other vegetables. Stay away from the following:

- Parsnips
- Sweet potatoes
- Potatoes

Drinks: The worst things to drink when following the keto diet are ones that have hidden sugar or are high in carbs. Here is a list of What You Need to avoid:

- Milkshakes
- Frappuccinos
- Smoothies (unless you make them yourself)
- Sodas
- Sweetened tea
- Vitamin water
- Energy drinks
- Orange juice
- Kombucha tea
- Caffe latte
- Beer
- Soy milk

- Milk
- Vegetable juice
- Coconut water

You might be getting rid of all the unwanted foods in your pantry, but these could feed other people. Please don't just throw these in the trash. Find a homeless shelter or local food pantry to give them to. You will be doing your community a service, plus you have a tax write off.

Go Shopping

Now that you have gotten rid of all the bad foods in your house, it is time to restock your freezer, refrigerator, and pantry with delicious foods that will help you feel great, get healthy and lose weight.

Poultry and meat: You get to eat lots of poultry and meat while following the ketogenic diet. These meats contain no carbs and have vitamin B and essential minerals like potassium, zinc, and selenium. You can eat any of the following meats:

- Deer
- Wild boar
- Bison
- Duck
- Goose
- Lamb
- Chicken
- Turkey
- Bacon
- Sausage
- Ham
- Steak
- Pork

- Beef

Eggs: Eggs are a great option when following a keto diet. They contain less than one gram of carbs and under five grams of protein. Eat them however you like them such as boiled, scrambled, fried, etc.

Healthy Fats: These are essential for the keto diet and should make up about 75 percent of your total calories. You can use the following fat sources:

- Seeds
- Nuts
- Eggs
- Meat fat
- Fatty fish
- Avocados
- Ghee
- Butter
- Full-fat dairy
- MCT oil
- Extra virgin olive oil
- Olive oil

Seafood and Fish: Fish is a great keto food. They are full of potassium, selenium, vitamin B, and contain almost no carbs. You can get your seafood and fish from the following sources:

- Prawn
- Crayfish
- Scallops
- Lobster
- Crabs
- Mussels

- Oysters
- Shrimp
- Trout
- Mahi-mahi
- Tuna
- Pollock
- Monkfish
- Skate
- Haddock
- Sea bass
- Catfish
- Tilapia
- Cod
- Mackerel
- Anchovies
- Sardines
- Salmon
- Clams

Vegetables: These are the foods that you need to eat the most of while following this diet as long as they are low carb. Vegetables contain fiber which helps you feel fuller longer. Here is a list of vegetables that you can consume:

- Carrots
- Green beans
- Brussels sprouts
- Peppers
- Kale

- Broccoli
- Cauliflower
- Cabbage
- Zucchini
- Cucumbers
- Eggplant
- Tomatoes
- Olives
- Asparagus
- Avocados
- Lettuce
- Spinach
- Celeriac
- Beets
- Onions

Dairy: You will need to eat these fats in moderation to follow the keto diet successfully. You can get quality fats from high-fat dairy. They also contain minerals, vitamins, and protein. These dairy sources are safe:

- Ricotta cheese
- Plain Greek yogurt
- Swiss cheese
- Cream cheese
- Sour cream
- Cream
- Blue cheese
- Mozzarella cheese

- Gouda cheese
- Cheddar cheese
- Ghee
- Butter
- Paneer
- Feta cheese
- Cottage cheese

Seeds and nuts: These are perfect for the keto diet because they are gut-friendly and dense in nutrients but these can only be eaten in moderation. Here are some seeds and nut sources:

- Seed milk
- Nut milk
- Sunflower seeds
- Sesame seeds
- Pumpkin seeds
- Hempseeds
- Flaxseeds
- Chia seeds
- Pistachios
- Walnuts
- Pecans
- Macadamia nuts
- Hazelnuts
- Cashews
- Brazil nuts
- Almonds

- Seed oil
- Nut oil

Spices and Seasonings: These are a good way to flavor your meals but you have to be careful as some spices do have some carbs but they shouldn't be a problem if you just learn to eat in moderation. Here is a list of seasonings and spices you can use:

- Oregano
- Thyme
- Rosemary
- Curry
- Nutmeg
- Cloves
- Ginger
- Turmeric
- Cumin
- Cinnamon
- Mustard seeds
- Cayenne pepper
- Chili powder
- Paprika
- Onion powder
- Garlic powder
- Black pepper
- Sea salt
- Cilantro
- Mint
- Basil

- Parsley

Fruits: There are only a few fruits you are allowed to eat while following the keto diet because they are low carb and low in sugar. These have to be eaten in moderation.

- Strawberries
- Blackberries
- Raspberries
- Blueberries
- Lemons
- Limes

The limes and lemons can be used to flavor water or drinks if needed.

Drinks: The following is a list of drinks that are best for you when following a keto diet:

- Tea and Coffee: You can still have your tea and coffee while on the ketogenic diet. Just be sure not to add in any sugar.

- Water: The best thing you can drink for your body is water. Water doesn't have any carbs and replenishes your body of the water it gets rid of. If you want more flavor for your water, try adding in some lemon or drink soda water. If you are going through the keto flu or are having headaches, add some salt to your water.

- Alcohol: You need to be careful when drinking alcohol because some have hidden sugars and carbs. The following alcohols are fine to drink in moderation:
    - Brandy
    - Tequila
    - Vodka
    - Cognac
    - Whiskey

Sweeteners: There are a few low carb natural sugar replacements. You will need to experiment and see what you like the taste of and what your body responds to. When you are having a sugar craving or want to take your coffee to the next level, it is nice to have something on hand to keep your sweet tooth under control and blood sugar stable.

- Stevia
- Erythritol

Getting the Kitchen Ready

Cooking delicious recipes is a great part of the keto diet. It is very easy if you have the correct tools. These tools will help make cooking faster and simpler. Everyone is worth the investment, especially if you cook a lot.

- *Food Scale*

When you are doing your best to reach your macronutrient and caloric goals, a food scale is a necessity. You have the ability to measure any liquid or solid foods and will have the perfect amount each time. If you use it in combination with apps such as MyFitnessPal, you will have the data you need to reach your goals. You can find food scales online for less than $20.

- *Food Processor*

These appliances are crucial for your kitchen arsenal. They are great for processing and blending specific foods together into shakes and sauces. Blenders won't cut it for most foods such as tough veggies like broccoli and cauliflower.

A great blender/processor is the NutriBullet. The containers you use to blend come with drink spouts or lids so you can take them on the go or use them for storage. They are easy to clean and make the entire system very convenient. You can usually find them for around $80 online.

- *Knife Sharpening Stone*

The majority of your time spent in the kitchen is on cutting. You will cut your chopping speed in half if you have a sharp knife. It is also pleasurable to use knives that are sharpened well. Try to sharpen your knives each week to keep them in great shape. Sharpening stones cost less than ten dollars and you can usually find them online. Most professional chefs will sharpen their knife before each use.

- *Spiralizer*

These fun little gadgets make vegetables into ribbons or noodles in just seconds. They make cooking easier and faster. Noodles have more surface area and only take half the time to cook. This gadget will turn zucchini into zoodles. Add in some marinara or Alfredo sauce and you will never know that you aren't eating actual pasta. Spiralizers can be found online and in most retail stores. They cost about $30.

- ***Cast Iron Pans***

These beauties have been used for centuries and were some of the first modern cooking utensils. They don't wear out and are healthy to use. They haven't been treated with any chemicals. They retain heat and can go between the stove top and the oven. They are an easy cleanup. All you need to do is wash them out using a non-scratch sponge and no soap, dry them, and rub them with some oil. This will prevent rust and helps keep them seasoned. Most pans will come pre-seasoned because this method will preserve the coating. They can be found online and in most retail stores. They generally cost between $10 and $80. It all depends on the size and brand. Lodge is still the most popular and continues to be made in the United States.

- ***Electric Hand Mixer***

If you have tried to beat an egg white by hand until they have formed stiff peaks, then you understand how hard this is. Electric hand mixers will save the muscles of your arm, especially if you are mixing heavy ingredients. It can also save you time. You can find good ones online or in retail stores for less than $20.

Meal Prep

Meal prep is the best way to do things if you want to save money, time, and make dieting super easy. Let's learn everything we can about meal prep.

Many people say the hard part of the ketogenic diet is following it. Meal prep can make this a lot easier. Think about a time you might have tried a diet but you didn't have access to meals. This is why most people turn to fast food places because it is easy and quick. Meal prep turns your refrigerator into a grab-it-and- go dispensary. To simply define meal prep would be the process of planning what you will be eating and how you will make it. The main purpose is saving yourself money and time.

The main part of this is planning and setting aside time to cook. This is a lot easier said than done. Putting forth the effort to plan ahead is going to save energy and time. It will also give you the results that you will be able to feel and see.

More importantly, meal prepping will help you with your dieting goals. It can help you discover the best you by helping you create a constant and healthy routine and stay away from the temptation of eating easy, quick, and unhealthy choices. Having prepped meals in your fridge for easy meals will work wonders for your goals and nutrition. It is hard to be successful when you are dieting as well as trying to maintain a healthy lifestyle since many foods require some sort of prep. We have been hardwired to take the easy route and choose what is
convenient and quick.

For some, meal prep might mean chopping veggies beforehand that gets cooked later. It might also mean measuring out ingredients before you start cooking.
Most people prepare the meals they will be eating for a whole week in one day and keep them stored in the refrigerator.

Begin Simple

The biggest part of meal prep is making sure it is stress-free and simple. There is no reason that meal prep has to be extravagantly made with ingredients that are complicated.

Meal Prep Ideas

There are several great ideas when meal prepping. Let's learn about the best ideas out there. You might have to experiment in your kitchen to figure out which way works best for you. This chapter should give you the inspiration you need to create your own meal prep layout.

- *Plan Ahead*

Since you are reading this book, you have likely already decided to try the ketogenic diet. The best way to begin this diet is to start with just a few recipes. You only need enough for one week. Find recipes that you like and make a plan.
Create a shopping list and take a trip to the grocery store to get What You Need to make these recipes.

- *Batch Cook*

If you are new to this diet and meal prep, don't let it intimidate you. This way of life is going to save you from stress during the week. Just sit down and plan ahead before you begin cooking. Be patient with yourself when you are trying to multitask in the kitchen. The more you learn to cook many things at one time, the better you will be.

- *Figure Out Your Rhythm*

You might find that you need to sit down with paper and pen and figure out what meals you want to cook. Keep in mind what foods will stay fresher longer along with what foods are on sale at which stores. Put your shopping list in order according to where they are located inside the store. When you have finished your shopping, sit down and figure out how you will attack the prep process. Think about ways to reuse pans or bowls whenever possible. Figure out if you can bake things simultaneously, and how you can make the most of your kitchen time.
Make sure you have enough time to allow the food to cool before you seal the containers and place them in the fridge.

- *Roast Veggies*

When you need to cook a lot of vegetables, try roasting them all at one time. You could roast a batch of veggies that cook quickly like mushrooms, cherry tomatoes, and asparagus. You could also make a batch of vegetables that roast slower like cauliflower, carrots, Brussels sprouts, and broccoli. These can now be stored and used later in the week. This helps reduce time lost and will help you maximum output.

Storage

Here's hoping that meal prep will be a normal routine for your house. For this to happen successfully, you have to choose and invest in the proper storage containers. You need to purchase a few various options like BPA-free plastic, metal, and glass. You can do trial runs to see what works best for you before making a large purchase. Try some and see what you like and what will save you money and time.

Plastic Containers

Quality containers are necessary to keep your food fresh for as long as you can. These are great for meal prep as they are lightweight, freezable, microwavable, and stacks easy. As stated above, be careful with plastics. Make sure they are BPA-free so you won't run the risk of making yourself or your family sick. Plastics aren't biodegradable. This means the earth can't absorb them back into the soil. Plastic can contaminate the soil. Unlike glass, plastics can absorb odors. Whatever you store might taste like what was stored before. Plastic remains cheaper than other storage options, but they don't last as long.

Sectioned Containers: Having these sectioned containers will be a lifesaver. These will give you the space you need to separate each item of the meal without them being mixed together. You can place the main course in the largest section with the sides in the smaller two. This makes it easy to grab out of the fridge and take with you to work or school to be heated up later.

BPA-free: By now, you have seen or read BPA-free on plastic items and this is why it is important. BPA are initials for bisphenol A. This is a chemical that is found in plastics such as consumer goods, food cans, water bottles, and food containers. Researchers say that BPA could seep into beverages and foods from the plastic containers that are made with BPA. There are some possible side effects to being exposed to BPA which include mental health problems, higher blood pressure, and negative effects on children, infants, and even fetuses.

Stackable: Everybody has a cabinet or drawer full of lids and containers. If you start making meal prep a regular routine, this means you are going to begin accumulating a lot of containers. Having stackable containers will keep your cabinets organized and functional and this will make your life a lot easier.

Freezer-safe: There are going to be times when you meal prep and have more food than what will be able to use in a week's time. This is why having freezer- safe containers is a necessity. You can also double recipes so you can put them in the freezer to be used later.

Dishwasher-safe: This one should be fairly obvious. Nobody wants to waste time having to hand wash dishes.

Microwave-safe: You are the only person who knows how you like to reheat your meals. Microwaving will be the most convenient. Choosing containers that are microwave-safe is another thing you need to pay attention to.

Glass Containers

Glass containers are great for several reasons. They are environmentally friendly. They are safe to use at various temperatures. This lets you reheat meals in the containers in the oven or microwave. Glass is a bit more expensive than plastic, but you get durability and safety. They also won't keep smells in them after cleaning. Circular, rectangular, or square containers can be found almost anywhere. You need to have a mixture of sizes for more versatility.

Lidded Jars

You need to have a variety of these versatile beauties around. You should try to have a several wide-mouth pint and quart jars along with some small four-ounce ones to hold sauces and dressings. They can be used to store healthy salads, snacks, sauces, and soups. Just layer your salad ingredients inside a jar. Don't put the dressing on it or it will get soggy. This is where those small jars come in
handy.

Stainless Steel

These last longer than plastics. Their appearance is nice and they hold cold and hot temperatures well. They are very durable. They are more expensive, and a drawback is metal can't be used in the microwave.

Skewers

When someone thinks about skewers, they automatically think kebabs. You can use wooden skewers as a measuring tool for veggies and meats. By doing this, you can cut meat for many skewers and divide them evenly. They can be stored for many days ahead of time. When it is time to cook, just take the meat off the skewers and cook them.

Freeze Smoothies in Muffin Tins

Muffin tins are very useful. To save some time each morning, pour your smoothie into muffin tins. This will save you time and gives you a great smoothie each day. Just take out a few cups, pop them in the blender and you have a healthy breakfast. Because they are frozen, you don't have to use water or ice.

Keep Records

It is a good idea to keep track of your accomplishments so you can look back on your achievements. Reaching milestones will give you the encouragement and inspiration to keep pushing forward until you've reached your goals.

Labeling

I used to not worry about labeling my foods as I prepped them until I realized how much I was throwing away. I thought I could remember when everything was bought and would use it before they went bad. Once you begin labeling and prepping meals, you will be more aware of what is in the refrigerator and when you need to use it and this will, in turn, save you money.

Keep a permanent marker and a roll of freezer tape in the kitchen. Label everything by putting a "best by" date on it so you know how long every meal is good for.

Thawing

The best way to thaw foods is to put them in the refrigerator. This does mean you have to think ahead and give yourself time for it to thaw in the refrigerator before you need it.

Using the cold water method could be quicker than the fridge method but this requires some attention. The food has to be in a bag that is leak-proof and completely under cold water. The water should be changed every half hour until it is thawed completely.

You should never freeze and thaw fish. It will last for four days in the fridge.

Reheating

Microwaving is the most popular and fastest way to reheat food. I normally try to reheat in one-minute intervals until it is at my desired temperature. Watch the food and stir it after each minute. This makes sure it reaches an even temperature all over.

You could also use your oven or grill to reheat, too. Another option would be using a skillet on the stovetop. You just simply empty the meal out into a skillet and stir until it has reached the correct temperature.

When you are reheating leftover, you need to get them to a temperature of 165.

Storage Tips

When you purchase dairy and meats, always look for products that have a "sell by" date that is the farthest away. It might mean you have to dig to the back but these foods will stay in storage longer.

Be sure your prepped meals have cooled completely before you put a lid on them and put them in the freezer or refrigerator. If you put the lid on while it is still hot, it is going to create steam that will cause the foods to continue to cook. This can cause proteins to become dry and veggies to be overcooked.

Mistakes to Avoid

Now that you understand how to meal prep, let's look at some common mistakes to avoid:

- Don't rush when cooking meals. Thinking about cooking an entire week's meals might seem a bit daunting, but you need to take your time. It is best to prep meals on the weekend or when you have a day off from work.

- Don't leave food on the counter too long or bacteria might begin forming. Once the food has cooled, you need to keep the food in a lidded container and in the refrigerator to lessen the chances of germs or bacteria setting in.

- Be sure you wash the containers along with their lids after each use. If you don't clean them properly, it could result in bacteria getting into your meals.

- Use fresh ingredients. It is best to prep meals when you get home from the store. If you use vegetables and meats that are old, you might find rotting foods in your refrigerator before you have time to enjoy the meal.

- When you are prepping salad, don't add the salad dressing in. This can cause your vegetables to become soggy. You can add the salad dressing on the bottom and place the protein on top of the dressing. Proteins won't get soggy. You could also put the dressing in a small jar and take it with you.

- Switch up recipes every week or so. This keeps you from getting tired of the same foods. The collection of keto recipes that can be found at the end of this book will make sure you are always excited when it comes time to eat.

- Heat your foods properly. Just be careful not to overheat them as this could cause the food to burn. It can also cause nutrients to become killed off in the reheating process. It could dry out the food where it becomes impossible to eat. If you don't heat it enough, it could leave bacteria in your food that will make you sick.

Meal Prep for Beginners

By now, you understand the basics of a ketogenic diet and meal prepping. As you can see, these two things go hand in hand. These meal prep plans are meant to help make your life easier and lower your stress. This first two-week meal prep plan is perfect for the beginner. It gives you an idea of what your meals should look like and gives you the perfect place to start. It will also slowly introduce you to intermittent fasting.

During the first week, you will have breakfast recipes that you get to enjoy. Then, as you transition into the second week, breakfast recipes will be replaced with keto coffee. Keto coffee doesn't require any prepping, but it only takes a few extra seconds in the morning so it won't ruin your day.

When you start out, the recipes may come off as a bit repetitive, but when you realize how much time you are saving by prepping and not having to constantly figure out your macros, it will be worth it. You will also find shopping lists, which are easy on the wallet. Once you have the big keto staples in your pantry, your shopping trips will cost less. Fats aren't all the same, so you may want to spend a few extra bucks for healthy fats like avocado oil and coconut oil.

The Recipes for WEEK ONE Are:

- Zoodle Chicken Parmesan

- Fajita Salad

- Zucchini Boats

- Breakfast Muffins

The Recipes for WEEK TWO Are:

- Keto Coffee

- Cobb Salad

- Bacon Cheese Burgers

- Chicken Salad Wraps

WEEK ONE Shopping List

Dairy:

- 8-ounce container sour cream
- Cheddar cheese
- Parmesan

Protein:

- 6-ounces cooked ham
- 3 Dozen egg
- 1 pound Italian sausage
- 2-pound flank steak
- 3 bone-in chicken thighs

Produce:

- Tomato
- Broccoli
- Green bell pepper
- Avocado
- 6 zucchinis
- 2 onions
- 3 limes
- 1 head romaine
- Cilantro

Pantry:

- Onion powder
- Garlic powder
- Dijon mustard
- Cooking spray
- Salt
- Red pepper flakes
- 2 cups pork rings
- Paprika
- Oregano
- 16- ounces Low-carb marinara sauce
- Extra-virgin olive oil
- Cumin
- Coconut oil
- 14.5-ounces chicken broth
- Pepper

Equipment:
- Baking sheet
- Baking dish
- Vegetable spiralizer
- 11 storage containers
- Skillet
- Mixing bowls
- Measuring spoons and cups
- Immersion blender
- Ice tray or silicone molds

- Cutting board
- Knife

Day One:
- Breakfast: Breakfast Muffins
- Lunch: Zoodle Chicken Parmesan
- Dinner: Fajita Salad

Day Two:
- Breakfast: Breakfast Muffins
- Lunch: Fajita Salad
- Dinner: Zucchini Boats

Day Three:
- Breakfast: Breakfast Muffins
- Lunch: Zucchini Boats
- Dinner: Zoodle Chicken Parmesan

Day Four:
- Breakfast: Breakfast Muffins
- Lunch: Fajita Salad
- Dinner: Zucchini Boats

Day Five:
- Breakfast: Breakfast Muffins
- Lunch: Zoodle Chicken Parmesan
- Dinner: Fajita Salad

WEEK ONE Prep

1. Marinate your flank steak.
2. Set your oven to 400.
3. Fix the breakfast muffins and slide them in your oven.
4. Check your breakfast muffins. Once the eggs are completely set, take them out of the oven. Set them aside to cool. Turn the oven to 375.
5. Work through the first four steps of the Zoodle Chicken Parmesan and get your zucchini noodles ready.
6. Work through step five for the Zucchini Boats.
7. In the same skillet you were using for the boats, get the peppers and onions ready for the fajita salad.
8. Check on your chicken, and once it has cooked through, take it out and allow it to cool. Turn the oven to 350 and work through step six of the Zucchini Boats recipe.
9. Once the boats are done, allow them to cool off before placing them in the storage containers.
10. Flip the oven to broiler and follow the second step of Fajita Salad. 11. Finish

up the chicken parmesan.

Breakfast Muffins

This recipe makes 5 servings and contains 364 calories; 23 g fat; 30 g protein; 7 g net carbs per serving

What You Need

- Dijon mustard, 1 tsp.
- Diced tomatoes, .5 c
- Shredded cheddar, 1 c
- Cubed ham, 1 c
- Chopped broccoli, 1.5 c
- Garlic powder, .5 tsp.
- Onion powder, .5 tsp.
- Pepper
- Salt
- Eggs, 15
- Cooking spray

What to Do

1. Heat up your oven to 400 and grease 15 cups on two muffin tin pans. You can also line them with papers or silicone liners.

2. Mix together the garlic powder, onion powder, pepper, salt, and eggs together.

3. Stir in the mustard, tomatoes, cheese, ham, and broccoli.

4. The egg mixture should be evenly poured to the muffin cups.

5. Allow the muffins to bake for 15 minutes. The eggs should be completely set. Allow the muffins to cool off.

6. Place three muffins in five different storage containers.

Fajita Salad

This recipe makes 4 servings and contains 893 calories; 60 g fat; 70 g protein; 11 g net carbs per serving

What You Need

For the Salad:

- Avocado
- Quartered limes, 2
- Shredded cheddar, .5 c
- Sour cream, .5 c
- Chopped romaine, 6 c
- Sliced red and green bell peppers
- Sliced onion
- EVOO, 2 tbsp.

For the Steak:

- Pepper
- Salt
- Chopped cilantro, 1 bunch
- Juice of a lime
- EVOO, .25 c
- Garlic powder, 1 tsp.
- Onion powder, 1 tsp.
- Cumin, 1 tsp.
- Flank steak, 2 lb.

What to Do

For the Steak:

1. Place the flank steak in a bag and add in the pepper, salt, cilantro, lime juice, cumin, onion powder, garlic powder, and oil. Shake everything together and marinate for no more than 24 hours.

2. Once you are ready to cook, flip the broiler on and lay the steak on a baking sheet. Discard the remaining marinade. Bake the steak for three to five minutes on both sides. Allow the steak to rest for at least ten minutes. Thinly slice the steak against the grain.

For the Salad:

1. Heat up a skillet and add in the peppers, onion, and oil. Stir the mixture often, and let it cook for eight to ten minutes, or until the onions turn translucent.

2. In four different storage containers, divide the steak, onions, and peppers. On the other side of the containers, add the cheese, sour cream, lettuce, and lime wedges. Before you serve, top the steak with a quarter of chopped avocado. Mix everything together and squeeze some lime juice over the top.

Zoodle Chicken Parmesan

This recipe makes 3 servings and contains 649 calories; 42 g fat; 45 g protein; 19 g net carbs per serving

What You Need

For Serving:

- Pepper
- Salt
- Low-carb marinara, 1.5 c
- Zucchini noodles, 3 c

For the Zoodles:

- Pepper
- Salt
- Minced garlic, 1 tsp.
- EVOO, 3 tbsp.s
- Zucchini, 4

For the Chicken:

- EVOO, 3 tbsp.
- Garlic powder, 1 tsp.
- Bone-in chicken thighs, 3
- Eggs, 2
- Pepper
- Salt
- Parmesan, .25 c
- Crushed pork rinds, 2 c

What to Do

For the Zoodles:

1. Use a spiralizer to turn the zucchini into noodles.

2. Add the oil to a skillet and cook the garlic for a minute.

3. Add in the zucchini and toss so that it becomes coated in the oil. Allow them to cook for two to five minutes, or until they become tender. Make

sure you don't overcook them because zucchini can quickly become mushy. You want them to have a bit of a crunch.

For the Chicken:

1. Start by placing your oven to 375.

2. Mix the parmesan and pork rinds together in a bowl and add in some pepper and salt. In another dish, beat the eggs.

3. Dry off the chicken and dip each one in the egg wash and then in the pork rind mixture.

4. Use a large pan made of cast iron to warm up the oil and add in the chicken thighs. Cook them for six to seven minutes on each side. Make sure that they cook completely on one side before moving or flipping.

5. Slide the chicken in the oven and let them finish cooking for 25-30 minutes. They should reach 165.

6. In three different containers, add in a c of zoodles, a half of a c of marinara, and a chicken thigh.

Zucchini Boats

This recipe makes 3 servings and contains 720 calories; 55 g fat; 44 g protein; 11 g net carbs per serving

What You Need

- Pepper
- Salt
- Parmesan, .75 c
- Chicken broth, 1 c
- Oregano, 2 tsp.
- Minced garlic, 2 tbsp.
- Ground Italian sausage, 1 lb.
- Paprika, 2 tsp.
- Red pepper flakes, 1 tsp.
- Diced onion
- Avocado oil, 1 tbsp.
- Zucchini, 3 – sliced lengthwise

What to Do

1. Heat your oven to 350.
2. Each zucchini half's flesh part should be scooped out using a spoon and then chopped.
3. Add the oil to a skillet and cook the sausage, garlic, and onion until the sausage has brown. This will take about six to eight minutes. Add in the oregano, red pepper flakes, paprika, and zucchini flesh.
4. Add equal portions of the sausage mixture to each of the zucchini shells. Place the zucchini boats in a baking dish and add the broth in the bottom.
5. Top the boats with parmesan and a shake of pepper and salt. Cook boats for 30-35 minutes. The cheese should be bubbly. Place two zucchini boats in each of three different storage containers.

WEEK TWO Shopping List

Dairy:

- 4-ounces blue cheese
- 4-ounces cheddar cheese
- 1-pint heavy cream
- Salted butter

Protein:

- 1 Dozen eggs
- 8-ounces bacon
- 1 ¼ pound skinless and boneless thighs of chicken
- 1 ½ pounds ground beef
- Mayonnaise

Produce:

- Onion
- Parsley
- 2 heads romaine lettuce
- Butter leaf lettuce
- Lemon
- 1 pint grape tomatoes
- Garlic
- 2 cucumbers
- Celery

Pantry:

- Worcestershire sauce
- Salt
- 24-ounces mayonnaise
- Full-fat coconut milk
- Pepper
- Avocado oil
- Apple cider vinegar

Equipment:
- Whisk
- 16 storage containers
- Muffin tin
- Mixing bowl
- Measuring spoons and cups
- Cutting board
- Knife
- 2 baking sheets

Day One:
- Breakfast: Keto Coffee
- Lunch: Bacon Cheese Burger
- Dinner: Cobb Salad

Day Two:
- Breakfast: Keto Coffee
- Lunch: Cobb Salad

- Dinner: Chicken Salad Wraps

Day Three:
- Breakfast: Keto Coffee
- Lunch: Cobb Salad
- Dinner: Chicken Salad Wrap

Day Four:
- Breakfast: Keto Coffee
- Lunch: Chicken Salad Wrap
- Dinner: Bacon Cheese Burger

Day Five:
- Breakfast: Keto Coffee
- Lunch: Bacon Cheese Burger
- Dinner: Cobb Salad

WEEK TWO Prep

1. Start by prepping the Bacon Cheese Burger patties and refrigerate them.
2. Hard-boil the eggs that you need for this week.
3. Place your bacon and chicken thighs on the two baking sheets.
4. Fix your Ranch dressing and place in the refrigerator.
5. Turn your oven to 375. Slide your bacon and chicken thighs in the oven.
6. Prep the celery, onions, cucumbers, and romaine for the Chicken Salad Wraps and Cobb Salad and place to the side.
7. Check on the things in the oven. Once they are both cooked through, drain the bacon on paper towels and allow the chicken to cool off. The chicken will take longer to cook than the bacon will.

8. Work through the first three steps of the Cobb Salad recipe.

9. Finish out the Bacon Cheese Burger recipe. 10. Pull together the Chicken Salad Wraps.

Ranch Dressing

This recipe makes 1 ½ cups, and contains 83 calories; 5 g net carbs per 2 tablespoons; <1 g protein; 7 g fat

What You Need

- Pepper
- Salt
- Mayonnaise, 1 c
- Full-fat coconut milk, .5c
- Minced garlic, 2 cloves
- Lemon juice, 1 tbsp.
- Apple cider vinegar, 1 tbsp.
- Chopped parsley, 2 tbsp.

What to Do

1. Use a blender to mix all of the ingredients together for one to two minutes, or until it becomes smooth. Taste, and add some pepper and salt if needed.

2. Pour this into a jar and keep in the refrigerator.

Cobb Salad

This recipe makes 4 servings and contains 545 calories; 38 g fat; 33 g protein; 20 g net carbs per serving.

What You Need

- Ranch dressing, .5 c
- Sliced hard-boil eggs, 4
- Crumbled blue cheese, .5 c
- Chopped cooked bacon, 4 slices
- Chopped onion, .5 c
- Diced cucumbers, 2
- Grape tomatoes, 1 c
- Chopped cooked chicken thighs, 2 c
- Chopped romaine, 2 heads
- Mayonnaise, 1 c

What to Do

1. Place the lettuce evenly in four storage containers.
2. Place the eggs, blue cheese, bacon, onion, cucumbers, tomatoes, and chicken evenly in the four containers on top of the lettuce.
3. Divide the ranch dressing into single-serving containers, two tablespoons per container.

Chicken Salad Wraps

This recipe makes 3 servings and contains 783 calories; 70 g fat; 32 g protein; 2 g net carbs per serving.

What You Need

- Butterhead lettuce, 8 leaves
- Pepper
- Salt
- Mayonnaise, 2 c
- Dijon mustard, 1 tbsp.
- Minced celery, 3 stalks
- Minced onion, 2 tbsp.
- Chopped hard-boil eggs, 6
- Chopped cooked chicken thighs, 1.5 c

What to Do

1. Mix together the mustard, onion, celery, eggs, and chicken. Mix in the mayonnaise. Add in some pepper and salt to your liking.

2. Place the lettuce and egg salad in three storage containers. When you are ready to eat, place the egg salad in the lettuce leaves and wrap up.

Bacon Cheese Burger

This recipe makes 4 servings and contains 772 calories; 6 g net carbs per serving; 61 g protein; 54 g fat.

What You Need

- Grape tomatoes, 1 c
- Chopped avocado
- Chopped romaine lettuce, 1 head
- Pepper
- Salt
- Eggs, 2
- Worcestershire sauce, 1 tbsp.
- Crumbled blue cheese, .5 c
- Crumbled cooked bacon, 4 slices
- Ground beef, 1.5 lbs.

What to Do

1. Mix together the eggs, Worcestershire sauce, blue cheese, bacon, and beef. Add in some pepper and salt. Shape the meat mixture into four patties. Cover them in saran wrap and allow them to refrigerate up to two hours.

2. Heat up your broiler or grill and place the patties on the cooking surface allow them to cook for four to five minutes on both sides. You can cook them to your desired level of doneness. Allow the patties to cool.

3. In four storage containers, add the tomatoes, avocado, and lettuce. Top this with a burger patty.

Keto Coffee

This recipe makes 1 serving and contains 276 calories; 31 g fat; <1 g protein; <1 g net carbs.

What You Need

- Fresh coffee, 8-oz.
- Butter, 1 tbsp.
- Coconut oil, 1 tbsp.
- Heavy cream, 1 tbsp.

What to Do

1. Add all of the ingredients to your blender and mix them together for 30 seconds to a minute. Everything should come together and turn a bit frothy.

Meal Prep for Performance

This next meal prep is designed for the active person. So often people will use going to the gym as an excuse for eating crap. While it may keep you from gaining weight, and you might drop a few pounds, this isn't the healthiest thing to do.

When you are a big gym buff it can be tough to find time to cook healthy meals. This is where keto meal prep comes in. This meal prep will help you to reduce body fat and maintain all of your lean muscle.

During these two weeks, you will find that the protein intake has been increased and dairy has been completely eliminated. Dairy will often cause inflammation for people. By reducing or eliminating dairy, you will often see a greater fat reduction. Really listen to your body during these two weeks. You may find that your body does better without dairy and higher protein intake. Also, it is safe to fast while training as long as you make sure you consume some protein close to your workouts.

The Recipes for WEEK ONE:

- Breakfast Pudding

- Spaghetti Squash with Roasted Chicken

- Bratwursts

- Broccoli Stir-Fry

The Recipes for WEEK TWO:

- Keto Coffee

- Salmon and Arugula Salad

- Spaghetti Squash with Bolognese

- Cabbage Stir-Fry

WEEK ONE Shopping List

Protein:

- 4 bone-in chicken thighs
- 1 pound bratwurst sausage
- 1.5 pounds sirloin steak

Produce:

- 4 pound spaghetti squash
- Onion
- Ginger
- 2 crowns broccoli

Pantry:

- Sesame oil
- 16 ounces sauerkraut
- Salt
- Pesto sauce
- Onion powder
- Hemp hearts
- Garlic powder
- Flaxseed
- Shredded coconut
- 5 ounce can full-fat coconut milk
- Coconut aminos
- Cinnamon
- 14.5 ounce chicken broth

- Chia seeds
- Pepper
- Avocado oil
- Sliced almonds
- Vanilla
- Stevia

Equipment:

- Pot
- Mixing bowls
- Measuring spoons and cups
- Cutting board
- Colander
- Knife
- Baking sheet
- Skillet
- 17 storage containers

Day One:

- Breakfast: Breakfast Pudding
- Lunch: Broccoli Stir-Fry
- Dinner: Bratwursts

Day Two:

- Breakfast: Breakfast Pudding
- Lunch: Bratwursts

- Dinner: Spaghetti Squash with Roasted Chicken

Day Three:
- Breakfast: Breakfast Pudding
- Lunch: Spaghetti Squash with Roasted Chicken
- Dinner: Broccoli Stir-Fry

Day Four:
- Breakfast: Breakfast Pudding
- Lunch: Broccoli Stir-Fry
- Dinner: Spaghetti Squash with Roasted Chicken

Day Five:
- Breakfast: Breakfast Pudding
- Lunch: Bratwursts
- Dinner: Broccoli Stir-Fry

WEEK ONE Prep

1. Start to marinate the beef for the Broccoli Stir-Fry.
2. Set your oven to 375 and work through steps two through five for the Spaghetti Squash with Roasted Chicken.
3. As the chicken is cooking, work through the first two steps of Breakfast Pudding.
4. Once your chicken is cooked through, take it out of the oven and let it cool. Turn the heat to 350.
5. After slicing the spaghetti squash in two, the seeds should be removed next. And then, place them on a baking sheet with the cut-side down. Let it bake for 45-50 minutes, or until soft. Once cooked, let it cool and shred the strands out with a fork.

6. Get the <u>Bratwursts</u> ready.

7. Heat up a skillet and boil water in a large pot. Work through the first five steps of Broccoli Stir-Fry.

8. Finish the last steps of Spaghetti Squash with Roasted Chicken.

Breakfast Pudding

This recipe makes 5 servings and contains 397 calories; 5 g net carbs per serving; 7 g protein; 39 g fat

What You Need

- Sliced almonds, .25 c
- Vanilla, 2 tsp.
- Cinnamon
- Salt
- Stevia, 3 tsp.
- Flaxseed, 3 tbsp.
- Shredded coconut, .25 c
- Hemp hearts, .25 c
- Chia seeds, 3 tbsp.
- Unsweetened coconut milk, 2 13.6-ounce cans

What to Do

1. Mix the cinnamon, salt, Stevie, flaxseed, chia seeds, hemp hearts, coconut, and coconut milk together in a pot. Allow this to come to a boil. Next, simmer this over low heat, whisking constantly, until it has thickened. This will take about eight to ten minutes.

2. Remove from the heat. The vanilla should be added next.

3. Divide the pudding between five mason jars and top them with sliced almonds.

Broccoli Stir-Fry

This recipe makes 4 servings and contains 588 calories; 4 g net carbs per serving; 54 g protein; 38 g fat

What You Need

For the Broccoli:

- Pepper
- Sesame oil, .25 c
- Minced garlic, 3 cloves
- Minced ginger, 1 tbsp.
- Coconut aminos, .25 c
- Avocado oil, 2 tbsp.
- Trimmed and separated broccoli, 2 crowns
- Salt, 1 tsp.

For the Marinade:

- Sliced sirloin steak, 1.5 lb.
- Pepper
- Salt
- Sesame oil, 2 tbsp.
- Garlic powder, 1 tsp.
- Onion powder, 1 tsp.
- Avocado oil, .25 c
- Coconut aminos, 6 tbsp.

What to Do

In a mixing container, combine together all the ingredients for the marinade. Add in the steak and toss. Make sure that the steak is completely coated. Allow the steak to marinate for at least 30 minutes.

For the Broccoli:

1. Fill up a pot halfway with water and add in a teaspoon of salt. Let this come to a boil.

2. Place the broccoli in the water and blanch for one to three minutes. Pour into a colander to drain. Rinse the broccoli with cold water so that it doesn't continue to cook. Place to the side.

3. Add the ginger, garlic, and avocado oil to a large skillet and let them all cook for 30 seconds.

4. Mix in the beef. Discard the marinade. Cook the beef, stirring constantly, for two to three minutes. Mix in the sesame oil, coconut aminos, and broccoli. Add in some pepper and salt. Continue to cook this mixture until the beef has reached your desired doneness.

5. Split this mixture between four storage containers.

Bratwursts

This recipe makes 4 servings and contains 525 calories; 42 g fat; 24 g protein; 8 g net carbs per serving

What You Need

- Pepper
- Salt
- Garlic powder, 1 tsp.
- Chicken broth, 1.5 c
- Sauerkraut, 16-ounces – drained
- Bratwurst, 1 lb.
- Sliced onion
- Avocado oil, 2 tbsp.

What to Do

1. Add the oil, bratwurst, and onion to a cast iron skillet. Allow this to cook for six to eight minutes, or until they get some color.

2. Mix in the pepper, salt, garlic powder, broth, and sauerkraut. Let this mixture simmer for 30-40 minutes. The sausages should be cooked all the way through.

3. In four containers, add a c of sauerkraut and one bratwurst.

Spaghetti Squash with Roasted Chicken

This recipe makes 4 servings and contains 361 calories; 6 g net carbs per serving; 18 g protein; 30 g fat

What You Need

- Pesto, .25 c
- Cooked spaghetti squash
- Pepper
- Salt
- EVOO, .25 c
- Garlic powder, 1 tsp.
- Onion powder, 1 tsp.
- Bone-in chicken, 4 3-ounce thighs

What to Do

1. Set your oven to 375.

2. Dry off the chicken thighs and lay them in a shallow dish.

3. Add in the onion powder, garlic powder, and oil, along with some pepper and salt. Mix everything and make sure that the chicken is coated.

4. On a baking sheet, lay the chicken out.

5. Bake the chicken for about thirty to forty minutes. Cook the chicken thoroughly until it reaches 165 degrees.

6. Toss the pesto and the cooked spaghetti squash together. Season it with some pepper and salt. Make sure that the squash is completely coated.

7. Place the noodles evenly in four containers and top each one with a thigh. Let everything cool off before you place on the lids.

WEEK TWO Shopping List

Protein:

- 3 4-ounce salmon fillets
- 2 ½ pounds ground beef

Produce:

- 4 pound spaghetti squash
- 4 scallions
- Onion
- Lemon
- Garlic
- Celery
- Head of cabbage
- Green bell pepper
- 8 ounces of arugula

Pantry:

- 14.5-ounce can diced tomatoes; low-sugar
- 6-ounce can tomato paste
- Salt
- Oregano
- Garlic salt
- Garlic powder
- Extra-virgin olive oil
- Coconut oil
- Coconut aminos
- Pepper
- Apple cider vinegar

Equipment:

- 11 storage containers
- Skillet
- Measuring cups and spoons
- Cutting board
- Knife
- Baking sheet baking dish

Day One:

- Breakfast: Keto Coffee or Fasting
- Lunch: Cabbage Stir-Fry
- Dinner: Salmon and Arugula Salad

Day Two:

- Breakfast: Keto Coffee of Fasting
- Lunch: Spaghetti Squash with Bolognese
- Dinner: Cabbage Stir-Fry

Day Three:

- Breakfast: Keto Coffee or Fasting
- Lunch: Salmon and Arugula Salad
- Dinner: Spaghetti Squash with Bolognese

Day Four:

- Breakfast: Keto Coffee or Fasting
- Lunch: Cabbage Stir-Fry
- Dinner: Salmon and Arugula Salad

Day Five:

- Breakfast: Keto Coffee of Fasting
- Lunch: Spaghetti Squash with Bolognese
- Dinner: Cabbage Stir-Fry

WEEK TWO Prep

1. Get the vegetables ready for the Spaghetti Squash with Bolognese and Cabbage Stir-Fry.

2. Set your oven to 450 and work through the first three steps of the Salmon and Arugula Salad.

3. Once the salmon is cooked through, take it out of the oven and lower the oven down to 350. Finish putting together the salmon salad.

4. Slice the spaghetti squash lengthwise and clean out the seeds. In a casserole dish, the squash should be laid with its cut-side down and pour water about a quarter inch. Allow the squash to cook for 45-50 minutes. Take the squash out of the oven and allow it to cool. With a fork, scrape out the strands from the squash.

5. Work through the first four steps of the Spaghetti Squash with Bolognese recipes.

6. Heat up your skillet and work through the first four steps of the Cabbage Stir-Fry recipe.

Cabbage Stir-Fry

This recipe makes 4 servings and contains 550 calories; 33 g fat; 49 g protein; 8 g net carbs per serving

What You Need

- Chopped scallions, 4
- Coconut aminos, 2 tbsp.
- Apple cider vinegar, 2 tbsp.
- Salt
- Pepper
- Chopped cabbage, 1 head
- Minced garlic, 2 cloves
- Ground beef, 1.5 lb.
- Coconut oil, 1 tbsp.

What to Do

1. In a skillet, the oil should be heated up before adding the garlic and beef. Brown the beef.

2. Add in the cabbage and let the mixture cook for eight to ten minutes more. The cabbage should wilt slightly.

3. Mix in the vinegar and coconut aminos. Season with a little bit of pepper and salt.

4. Divide the stir-fry between four storage containers. Serve the stir-fry with some scallions. You can also top it with some toasted sesame oil, sriracha, and sesame seeds if you want.

Spaghetti Squash with Bolognese

This recipe makes 4 servings and contains 415 calories; 24 g fat; 33 g protein; 18 g net carbs per serving

What You Need

- Cooked spaghetti squash
- Pepper
- Diced tomatoes, 14.5-ounce can – drained
- Erythritol, 1 tbsp.
- Oregano, 1 tbsp.
- Garlic powder, 1 tsp.
- Salt
- Tomato paste, 2 tbsp.
- Ground beef, 1 lb.
- Chopped bell pepper
- Chopped celery, 2 stalks
- Chopped onion
- EVOO, 1 tbsp.

What to Do

1. Add the oil to a skillet. Mix in the bell pepper, celery, and onion. Cook them, stirring often, for six to eight minutes. Once the vegetables have cooked, mix in the ground beef. Cook until the meat is thoroughly cooked.

2. Add in the pepper, salt, garlic powder, oregano, erythritol, tomatoes, and tomato paste. Boil the mixture before simmering it for 20-30 minutes. Stir the mixture occasionally.

3. Allow the sauce to cool.

4. Place the cooked spaghetti squash in equal amounts in four containers and top each of them with the Bolognese.

Salmon and Arugula Salad

This recipe makes 3 servings and contains 393 calories; 4 g net carbs per serving; 26 g protein; 31 g fat

What You Need

- Arugula, 4.5 c
- Juice of a lemon
- Garlic salt, 1 tsp.
- EVOO, 5 tbsp. – divided
- Salmon, 3 4-ounce fillets

What to Do

1. Set your oven to four hundred and fifty degrees. On a baking sheet, place the foil.

2. Rub the salmon fillets with two tablespoons of oil and season with the garlic salt. Lay the salmon on the baking sheet and drizzle the lemon juice over top of them.

3. Bake the salmon for 8-12 minutes, or until it flakes easily. Allow the salmon to rest for ten minutes.

4. In three containers, add 1.5 cups of arugula and season with some pepper and salt. Top with the salmon. When you are ready to eat, drizzle with a tablespoon of oil and toss everything together.

Meal Prep for Maintenance

After you have achieved your weight loss goals, keeping that weight off tends to be the hardest part. With this meal prep, your protein and calories will be upped, but your carbohydrate intake will remain low. When you hit the maintenance period, keeping your carbs low is still the most important thing. Calories and protein intake don't have to be stressed over as much.

Your body now runs on fat, so you can play around and see how your body works in ketosis. If you do want to try out some more carbs, pick sources that are unprocessed. Carbs are best consumed right after you have exerted a lot of energy. Stay far away from processed or refined carbs, though. Make sure you listen to what your body has to say. Give your body the carbs that it wants.

Recipes for WEEK ONE:

- Frittata

- Chili

- Salmon Salad

- Meatloaf with Green beans

Recipes for WEEK TWO:

- Keto Coffee

- Chicken Legs with Rice

- Taco Salad

- Caesar Salad

WEEK ONE Shopping List

Dairy:

- Parmesan
- 1 pint heavy cream
- Crumbled feta cheese
- Shredded cheddar

Protein:

- 1 pound sausage
- 4 6-ounce salmon fillets
- 8 ounces ground pork
- Dozen eggs
- 1 pound ground beef
- 8 ounces bacon

Produce:

- Spinach
- Scallions
- 1 pint raspberries
- Mixed greens
- 1 pound green beans
- Celery
- 6 ounces broccoli florets
- Red bell pepper

Pantry:

- Worcestershire sauce
- Walnuts
- 16 ounce can tomato paste
- 15-ounce can diced tomatoes
- Salt
- Pork rinds
- Pecans
- Ketchup
- 4-ounce can diced green chiles
- Garlic salt
- EVOO
- Erythritol
- Cumin
- Chili powder
- Coconut oil
- Pepper
- 14.5 ounce can beef broth
- Apple cider vinegar
- Mustard

Equipment:

- 18 storage containers
- Slow cooker
- Skillet
- Mixing bowls
- Measuring spoons and cups

- Cutting board
- Knife
- Baking sheet

Day One:
- Breakfast: Breakfast Frittata
- Lunch: Salmon Salad
- Dinner: Meatloaf with Green Beans

Day Two:
- Breakfast: Breakfast Frittata
- Lunch: Chili
- Dinner: Meatloaf with Green Beans

Day Three:
- Breakfast: Breakfast Frittata
- Lunch: Chili
- Dinner: Salmon Salad

Day Four:
- Breakfast: Breakfast Frittata
- Lunch: Salmon Salad
- Dinner: Chili

Day Five:
- Breakfast: Breakfast Frittata
- Lunch: Salmon Salad

- Dinner: Meatloaf with Green Beans

WEEK ONE Prep

1. Set your oven to 400 and work through steps one through five for the <u>Meatloaf with Green Beans</u>. Clean out the bowl and reuse it for the <u>Frittata</u>.

2. Using a cast iron skillet, cook the meats for the <u>chili</u>. First, brown the ground beef, and then set to the side. Next, cook the bacon, and set to the side. Finally, brown up the sausage for the frittata and the chili.

3. Prep all of the fresh produce for the Frittata and the celery for the chili. Place to the side.

4. Check the meatloaf and once it is cooked through, take out of the oven and allow it to cool. Lower the heat of the oven to 375.

5. Work through the first two steps for the Chili.

6. In the skillet you used for the meats, work through steps three through six for the Frittata.

7. Boil water and a dash of salt to a large pot. Add in the green beans and cook them for three to four minutes. Drain off the beans and place them in ice water to stop the cooking. Drain and follow the sixth step of the Meatloaf recipe. Place a square of butter on top of the beans in their containers.

Frittata

This recipe makes 5 servings and contains 392 calories; 31 g fat; 23 g protein; 5 g net carbs per serving

What You Need

- Thinly sliced scallions, 3
- Shredded cheddar, .5 c – divided
- Pepper
- Salt
- Heavy cream, 2 tbsp.
- Beaten eggs, 8
- Spinach, 2 c
- Chopped red bell pepper
- Chopped broccoli florets, 1 c
- Ground sausage, 8 oz.

What to Do

1. Set your oven to 375.
2. Add the sausage to a cast iron skillet and brown for four to five minutes. Take the sausage out of the skillet and drain off all but a tablespoon of fat.
3. Put the bell pepper, spinach, and broccoli to the skillet and cook until the spinach wilts. This will take about two to three minutes. Mix the sausage back in.
4. Whisk the cream and eggs together with some pepper and salt. Pour the eggs over the sausage mixture. Stir in a quarter c of cheddar cheese until everything is combined.
5. Slide this into the oven. Bake for about half hour. The tops should be browned. Take the frittata out of the oven and top with the rest of the cheese. Put this under the broiler until the cheese has melted and crisped up.
6. Allow the frittata to cool and then slice it into five equal wedges. Place each wedge into five storage containers. Sprinkle on the scallions.

Meatloaf with Green Beans

This recipe makes 4 servings and contains 481 calories; 27 g fat; 49 g protein; 10 g net carbs per serving

What You Need

- Blanched green beans, 3 c
- Erythritol, 1 tbsp.
- Apple cider vinegar, 1 tbsp.
- Ketchup, .25 c
- Pepper
- Salt
- Mustard, 1 tsp.
- Heavy cream, .25 c
- Parmesan, .25 c
- Crushed pork rinds, .5 c
- Egg
- Ground pork, 8 oz.
- Ground beef, 8 oz.

What to Do

1. 400 degrees should be your oven's temperature. On a baking sheet, place a foil.
2. Mix together the mustard, cream, parmesan, pork rinds, egg, pork, and beef. Add in some pepper and salt.
3. Form the meat into a loaf shape and place it on the baking sheet.
4. Mix together the erythritol, vinegar, and ketchup. Brush this over the meatloaf.
5. Slide this into the oven. Bake for thirty-five to forty minutes. Ensure it has a temperature of 160 degrees.
6. Allow the meatloaf to cool before slicing it into four equal pieces.
7. Place ¾ of a c of green beans and a slice of meatloaf into four storage containers.

Salmon Salad

This recipe makes 4 servings and contains 456 calories; 34 g fat; 36 g protein; 7 g net carbs per serving

What You Need

- Crumbled feta, .25 c
- Fresh berries, .25 c
- Salad greens, 4 c
- Erythritol, 1 tbsp.
- Coconut oil, 1 tbsp.
- Whole pecans, .5 c
- Pepper
- Salt
- EVOO, 2 tbsp.
- Salmon fillets, 4 6-oz. fillets

What to Do

1. Preheat your broiler and line a cooking sheet with foil.
2. Use olive oil to rub the salmon. Drizzle with some pepper and salt. Lay them on the cooking sheet and allow them to broil for 8-12 minutes. The salmon should easily flake with a fork.
3. Take the salmon out and set to the side.
4. Meanwhile, add the erythritol, coconut oil, and pecans to a skillet. Stir until the erythritol has dissolved and the pecans have become fragrant. This will take three to five minutes. Take the pecans out of the skillet and set to the side.
5. Toss together the feta, berries, and greens in a large bowl.
6. Using four storage containers, add a heaping c of salad mix in each and top with a salmon fillet and two tablespoons of pecans.

Chili

This recipe makes 5 servings and contains 629 calories; 37 g fat; 46 g protein; 20 g net carbs per serving

What You Need

- Worcestershire sauce, 1 tbsp.
- Chili powder, 1 tbsp.
- Cumin, 1 tbsp.
- Garlic salt, 1 tsp.
- Pepper, 1 tsp.
- Shredded cheese
- Sour cream
- Diced green chiles, 4 oz.
- Tomato paste, 6 oz.
- Diced tomatoes with juices, 15 oz.
- Chopped celery, 1 c
- Beef broth, 1 c
- Cooked ground sausage, 8 oz.
- Diced cooked bacon, 8 oz.
- Cooked ground beef, 8 oz.

What to Do

1. Add everything except for the sour cream and shredded cheese to a crock pot. Mix everything together. Set the cooker to high for four to six hours, or you can set it to low for eight to ten hours.

2. Allow the chili to cool off and then divide evenly into five containers. Serve with some sour cream and cheese.

WEEK TWO Shopping List

Dairy:

- 8 ounce sour cream
- Salted butter
- Parmesan
- Heavy cream
- Cheddar cheese

Protein:

- Dozen eggs
- 12 ounces boneless skinless chicken thighs
- 6 chicken legs
- Pound ground beef

Produce:

- 2 limes
- Head romaine
- Lemon
- 1 pint grape tomatoes
- Garlic
- Head cauliflower
- Head cabbage
- 2 onions

Pantry:

- Mustard

- Worcestershire sauce
- Taco seasoning
- Low-carb salsa
- Onion powder
- Garlic salt
- EVOO
- 16 ounce can black olives
- 14.5 ounce can beef broth
- Anchovy paste

Equipment:

- 3 storage containers
- Skillet
- Mixing bowl
- Measuring spoons and cups
- 7 16-ounce mason jars
- Cutting board
- Knife

Day One:

- Breakfast: Keto Coffee or Fasting
- Lunch: Taco Salad
- Dinner: Chicken Legs with Rice

Day Two:

- Breakfast: Keto Coffee of Fasting

- Lunch: Caesar Salad
- Dinner: Taco Salad

Day Three:
- Breakfast: Keto Coffee or Fasting
- Lunch: Chicken Legs with Rice
- Dinner: Caesar Salad

Day Four:
- Breakfast: Keto Coffee or Fasting
- Lunch: Caesar Salad
- Dinner: Taco Salad

Day Five:
- Breakfast: Keto Coffee of Fasting
- Lunch: Caesar Salad
- Dinner: Chicken Legs with Rice

WEEK TWO Prep

1. Set your oven to 375. Rub the chicken thighs with onion and garlic powder, pepper, and salt. Bake the chicken for twenty to thirty minutes.
2. Boil a pot of water and cook the eggs.
3. Work through the first step of <u>Taco Salad</u>.
4. As the chicken and beef are cooking, prep your cauliflower rice.
5. Once the chicken thighs are cooked through, remove and allow to cool. Once the ground beef is browned, allow it to cool as well.
6. Get the ingredients for the Taco Salad and <u>Caesar Salad</u> prepared.
7. Work through steps four through seven for the <u>Chicken Legs</u>.

8. As the chicken is cooking, put together the salads. Work through the first two steps for the Caesar Salad and the second step for the Taco Salad.

9. Once the chicken legs are cooked through, place them on a plate and allow to cool. Follow steps one through three of Chicken Legs with Rice to prepare the rice.

10. Once everything has cooled, divide the rice and chicken legs between four containers.

Caesar Salad

This recipe makes 4 servings and contains 586 calories; 6 g net carbs per serving; 33 g protein; 50 g fat

What You Need

- Chopped romaine, 1 head
- Chopped cooked chicken thighs, 2 c
- Parmesan, .5 c
- Sliced hard-boil eggs, 4
- Thinly sliced onion, .5 c
- Grape tomatoes, 1 c
- Low-carb Caesar dressing, .75 c

What to Do

1. Add three tablespoons of dressing to the bottom of four mason jars.

2. Next, add in the tomatoes, onion, eggs, cheese, and chicken. Top with the lettuce. When you are ready to eat, shake everything together and enjoy.

Taco Salad

This recipe makes 3 servings and contains 931 calories; 65 g fat; 57 g protein; 22 g net carbs per serving

What You Need

- Lime wedges, 2 limes
- Shredded cabbage, 1 head
- Shredded cheddar, .75 c
- Sliced black olives, 16 ounces
- Grape tomatoes, 1 c
- Low-carb salsa, .75 c
- Beef broth, .5 c
- Taco seasoning, .25 c
- Ground beef, 1 lb.

What to Do

1. Add the ground beef to a skillet and cook until browned through. This will take about seven to ten minutes. After adding the taco seasoning and the broth, simmer it until it has thickened, about three to five minutes. Make sure that beef has cooled completely before making the salad.

2. Using three mason jars, divide out the salsa, sour cream, tomatoes, olives, cheese, beef, cabbage, and a lime wedge. It needs to be layered in that order. When you are ready to eat, squeeze in the lime juice and shake the salad together.

Chicken Legs with Rice

This recipe makes 3 servings and contains 502 calories; 35 g fat; 34 g protein; 10 g net carbs per serving

What You Need

- Pepper
- Chicken legs, 6
- Onion powder, 1 tbsp.
- Garlic salt, 1 tbsp.
- Salt
- Shredded cheddar, .5 c
- Heavy cream, .5 c
- Uncooked cauliflower rice, 3 c
- Salted butter, 4 tbsp. – divided
- Chopped onion

What to Do

1. Cook the onion in two tablespoons of butter in a large skillet. The onions should become translucent. This will take about five minutes.

2. Mix in the cauliflower, and let it cook for five minutes.

3. Stir in the cream cheese along with some pepper and salt. Mix until the cheese has melted. This will take about two to three minutes. Pour this into another dish and allow it to cool off.

4. Using the same skillet, add in the reaming butter.

5. Rub the chicken with the pepper, garlic salt, and onion powder.

6. For fifteen minutes, cook the chicken in a pan. Turn the meat frequently. The skin should be golden and has reached 165.

7. Using three storage containers, add in a c of rice and two chicken legs.

Breakfast

Breakfast Casserole

This recipe makes 12 servings and contains 285 calories; 23 g fat; 17 g protein; 2 g net carbs per serving

What You Need

- Shredded Swiss cheese, 1 c
- Pepper
- Salt, .5 tsp.
- Heavy cream, 1 c
- Beaten eggs, 9
- Chopped onion
- Bulk breakfast sausage, 1 lb.

What to Do

1. Set your oven to 350 and grease a 9" x 13" casserole dish.
2. Add the sausage to a skillet and cook. Crumble up the sausage as it cooks. Allow it to brown up. This will take about five minutes.
3. Mix in the onions. Cook for two to three more minutes, or until the onions soften. Set this off of the heat.
4. As the sausage cools off, beat together the pepper, salt, cream, and eggs.
5. Fold the cheese and sausage into the eggs.
6. Spread the mixture into your greased casserole dish.
7. Slide this into the oven and allow it to back for an hour.
8. Cool the casserole slightly before you slice it into 12 pieces.
9. If meal prepping, place a square of the casserole into 12 storage containers. 10.
These will keep for five days in the refrigerator or for six months in the freezer. To reheat, place them in the oven at 350 for 20 minutes. You can also thaw in the fridge and microwave for a couple of minutes.

Breakfast Pizza

This recipe makes 4 servings and contains 644 calories; 47 g fat; 43 g protein; 10 g net carbs per serving

What You Need

- Halved cherry tomatoes, 8
- Shredded mozzarella, .5 c
- Red pepper flakes
- Oregano, 1 tsp.
- Heavy cream, .25 c
- Beaten eggs, 8
- Sliced mushrooms, 1 c
- Chopped onion, .5
- Cubed pancetta, 8 oz.
- Unsalted butter, 2 tbsp.

What to Do

1. Heat up your broiler and move the rack to the highest position.

2. Using an ovenproof pan, add the butter and cook until it starts to bubble. Add in the pancetta, stirring occasionally, until it turns brown. This will take about three to five minutes.

3. Mix in the mushrooms and onion. Stir often. Cook for three mins or until the vegetables become soft. Spread this across the bottom of the pan.

4. Whisk the red pepper flakes, oregano, cream, and eggs together. Pour the mixture into the hot pan. Cook the eggs, without stirring them, so that they set around the edges. To pull back the eggs' edges, use a spatula. Tilt the eggs and let the uncooked eggs to run into the empty spot. Cook until the edges have set up again.

5. Sprinkle the eggs with the cheese and then top with the tomatoes. Slide the frittata in the oven under the broiler and cook until the cheese has melted and browned. This will take about three to five minutes.

6. Allow the frittata to cool and then slice it into four wedges.

7. For meal prepping, place a wedge of the frittata into four storage containers.

8. These will keep for five days in the fridge or for six months in the freezer. Allow them to rest in the fridge overnight to thaw and then microwave for

a couple of minutes. You can also heat them in the oven at 375 for five to ten minutes.

Baked Eggs in Avocado

This recipe makes 6 servings and contains 613 calories; 6.07 g net carbs per serving; 21 g protein; 56 g fat

What You Need

- Pepper
- Salt
- Shredded cheddar, 6 tbsp.
- Eggs, 6
- Lime juice, 4 tbsp.
- Avocados, 3

What to Do

1. Start by placing your oven to 450.
2. Carefully slice open each avocado, remove the pit and some of the flesh.
3. Put the avocados onto a baking sheet. Brush each half with lime juice.
4. Crack one egg into each avocado half.
5. Season with pepper and salt.
6. Put into the oven and bake for ten minutes.
7. Carefully remove from oven and sprinkle with cheese. Bake for another two to three minutes to melt the cheese.
8. Using six storage containers, add one avocado. Cool completely before placing into the refrigerator.
9. This will keep for three days in the refrigerator. This won't freeze well because of the avocado.

Ham and Cheese Waffles

This recipe makes 6 servings and contains 538 calories; 1.33 g net carbs per serving; 46 g protein; 39 g fat

What You Need

- Basil, .5 tsp.
- Chopped ham, .25 c
- Baking powder, 1 tsp.
- Pepper, .25 tsp.
- Salt, .5 tsp.
- Paprika, .5 tsp.
- Shredded cheddar, .25 c
- Melted butter, .75 c
- Eggs, 8

What to Do

1. Using two bowls, separate the whites and yolks of four eggs. Keep the other four eggs to the side.
2. Into the bowl holding the egg yolks, add in the baking powder, butter, and salt. Whisk until thoroughly combined.
3. Fold in the cheese and ham, gently.
4. Into the bowl holding the egg whites, whisk these until stiff peaks form.
5. Place half the whites into the yolk mixture, fold gently, and let sit for a few minutes.
6. After adding in the remaining egg whites, fold to incorporate.
7. Add some batter to a greased waffle maker. Cook for four minutes.
8. Continue with the rest of the batter until all is used up.
9. Using six storage containers, add a waffle into each. Cool completely before closing.
10. These can be frozen for up to six months or kept in the refrigerator for five days.

Bacon, Egg, and Cheese Casserole

This recipe makes 8 servings and contains 307 calories; 37.8 g fat; 25.5 g protein; 4.1 g net carbs per serving

What You Need

- Pepper
- Salt
- Chopped green onions, 3
- Minced garlic, 2 cloves
- Chopped onion, 1
- Heavy whipping cream, .5 c
- Sour cream, .75 c
- Shredded cheddar, 1.5 cups
- Eggs, 12
- Sliced bacon, 12

What to Do

1. Start by placing your oven at 350.
2. Put the bacon into a skillet and cook until crispy. When cooked, put onto paper towels to drain. Once drained and cooled a bit, crumble into bits.
3. Add the pepper, salt, whipping cream, sour cream, and eggs into a bowl. Whisk until thoroughly incorporated.
4. Grease a 9" x 13" casserole dish with olive oil. Add the shredded cheese onto the bottom and spread until even.
5. Pour the egg mixture on top and then top with the bacon bits.
6. Wrap the top with aluminum foil.
7. Put into the oven and bake for 35 minutes until the edges are browned and the middle is set.
8. Take out of the oven. Garnish with green onions.
9. Cut into eight equal pieces.
10. Using eight storage containers, add in one portion per container.

11. This will keep for five days in the refrigerator. You can also freeze it up to six months. To reheat, allow it thaw in the fridge and microwave for a few minutes.

Blackberry Egg Bake

This recipe makes 4 servings and contains 163 calories; 1 g net carbs per serving; 9.83 g protein; 12 g fat

What You Need

- Salt
- Zest of one orange
- Coconut or almond flour, 4 tbsp.
- Vanilla, .25 tsp.
- Melted butter, 1 tbsp.
- Chopped rosemary, 1 tsp.
- Grated ginger, 1 tsp.
- Blackberries, .5 c
- Eggs, 6

What to Do

1. Start by placing your oven at 350.
2. Take four ramekins and grease them with olive oil.
3. Add salt, orange zest, coconut flour, ginger, butter, vanilla, and eggs into a bowl. Stir until combined. The batter should be smooth.
4. Add in rosemary and stir to combine.
5. Evenly divide the batter into the four ramekins.
6. Put the ramekins onto a baking sheet and divide the blackberries evenly among the ramekins.
7. Place the baking sheet into the oven and bake for 20 minutes until eggs are done.
8. Carefully remove from oven and let cool slightly before serving.
9. Let the ramekins cool completely. Gently remove from ramekins and place into four storage containers.
10. These can be frozen for six months or refrigerated for five days.

Mushroom and Sausage Frittata

This recipe makes 6 servings and contains 388 calories; 3.47 g net carbs per serving; 29 g protein; 16 g fat

What You Need

- Butter, 1 tbsp.
- Salt, .5 tsp.
- Pepper, .5 tsp.
- Paprika, .25 tsp.
- Basil, .5 tsp.
- Greek yogurt, .5 c
- Chopped onion, 1 medium
- Sliced mushrooms, 1 c
- Shredded cheddar, 1 c
- Chopped kale, 6 oz.
- Eggs, 12
- Breakfast sausage, 1 lb.

What You Need

1. Start by placing your oven to 350.
2. Place a large ovenproof skillet onto your stove and warm on medium heat.
3. Put the sausage into the skillet and cook until done or no longer pink. Spoon it out onto paper towels and let drain. Set to the side.
4. Add butter into the same skillet and melt. When melted, add the mushrooms and onions into the skillet. Sauté until the onions are translucent. Stir frequently. Remove and set to the side.
5. Put the basil, paprika, pepper, salt, yogurt, and eggs into a large bowl. Whisk until completely combined.
6. Add in the onion, mushrooms, half of the cheese, kale, and sausage. Stir again to combine everything.
7. Add more butter and pour this mixture into the same skillet. Cook on medium heat. Cook for four minutes. Do not stir.
8. Take off from the heat and sprinkle on the rest of the cheese.

9. Bake in the oven until the center is done or for about thirty minutes. Take out of the oven and let it cool for a few minutes before slicing.

10. Slice into six equal triangles and place into six storage containers. 11. This can be refrigerated for five days or frozen for six months.

Spinach and Leek Eggs

This recipe makes 6 servings and contains 238 calories; 5.7 g net carbs per serving; 13 g protein; 18 g fat

What You Need

- Shredded cheddar, 1.5 c
- Eggs, 6
- Minced garlic, 2 cloves
- Chopped leeks, 2
- Spinach, 1 c
- Pepper, .25 tsp.
- Salt, .25 tsp.
- Chili powder, 1 tsp.
- Coconut oil, 2 tbsp.

What to Do

1. Start by placing your oven to 425.

2. Place a skillet on medium heat onto the stove and warm. Melt the coconut oil.

3. Put in the spinach, garlic, and leeks. Sauté for eight minutes until soft.

4. The eggs should be cracked in a bowl. Add in the chili powder, pepper, salt, and cheese. Stir to combine.

5. Pour into skillet and scramble the eggs until the desired doneness.

6. Using six storage containers divide evenly and allow to cool completely before placing into the refrigerator for five days or freeze for six months.

Chorizo Bake

This recipe makes 4 serving, and contains 432 calories; 37 g fat; 26 g protein; 5.07 g net carbs per serving

What You Need

- Pepper
- Salt
- Chopped bell pepper, 1
- Chopped onion, 1 small
- Sliced bacon, 2
- Chopped chorizo sausage, 6 oz.
- Sour cream, 2 tbsp.
- Almond milk, 2 tbsp.
- Eggs, 4
- Coconut oil, 1 tbsp.

What to Do

1. You need to warm your oven to 350.

2. Over medium heat, warm a large skillet on the stove. Cook the bacon. Make sure it is crispy. Drain the bacon onto paper towels after removing from the skillet.

3. Add coconut oil to skill and let it melt. Add in bell pepper and onion. Cook for six minutes until slightly browned.

4. Add in the chorizo and continue to cook.

5. Place the sour cream, almond milk, and eggs into a large bowl and whisk until combined. Season with pepper and salt.

6. Pour into skillet and lower heat. Sprinkle with bacon and let it cook until the center is set.

7. Cut into four servings.

8. Using four storage containers, add one section into each container. Refrigerate for five days or freeze for six months.

Mushroom and Spinach Muffins

This recipe makes 12 servings and contains 173 calories; 13 g fat; 4.2 g protein; .8 g net carbs per serving

What You Need

- Italian seasoning, .5 tsp.
- Garlic powder, 1 tsp.
- Pepper
- Salt
- Chopped spinach, 2 c
- Chopped mushrooms, 1 c
- Coconut milk, .5 c
- Shredded cheese, 1 c
- Eggs, 8

What to Do

1. You need to warm your oven to 350.
2. Grease a muffin tin with olive oil.
3. Into a bowl, add in the garlic powder, Italian seasoning, pepper, salt, coconut milk, cheddar cheese, and eggs. Whisk to combine.
4. Add in the spinach and mushrooms.
5. Divide this mixture out into the muffin tin.
6. For twenty minutes, bake in the preheated oven until thoroughly cooked.
7. Take out of the oven and let cool.
8. For food prep, allow to cool completely and place into individual storage containers for five days or freeze for six months.

Lemon Poppy Pancakes

This recipe makes 4 servings and contains 378 calories; 5 g net carbs per serving; 31.3 g protein; 27.1 g fat

What You Need

- Erythritol, .25 c
- Liquid stevia, 10 drops
- Salt, .25 tsp.
- Coconut flour, .5 c
- Protein powder, 1 scoop
- Poppy seeds, 2 tbsp.
- Baking powder, 1 tsp.
- Heavy cream, 1 tbsp.
- Ricotta, 6 oz.
- Eggs, 6
- Zest and juice of 2 lemons

What to Do

1. In a food processor or blender, put the juice and zest of one lemon, stevia, eggs, and ricotta. Process until smooth.

2. Pour into a large bowl. Add in the protein powder, flour, poppy seeds, salt, and baking powder. Stir to combine.

3. Put a large nonstick skillet onto the stove and warm on medium heat.

4. Place about one-fourth c of the batter into the skillet.

5. Cook until bubble form on top and sides are set. Gently turn over and cook on the other side until browned.

6. Place onto plates and continue with batter until all is gone.

7. In another bowl, put the zest and juice of the other lemon, erythritol, and heavy cream. Whisk until combined.

8. Drizzle this lemon glaze over pancakes and enjoy.

9. Place any uneaten pancakes into a storage container and place into the freezer for up to six months or in the fridge for three days.

Coconut Blueberry Porridge

This recipe makes 4 servings and contains 392 calories; 11.53 g net carbs per serving; 11 g protein; 21 g fat

What You Need

- Ground flaxseed, .5 c
- Blueberries, 1 c
- Ground cinnamon, 1 tsp.
- Ground nutmeg, .5 tsp.
- Vanilla, 1 tsp.
- Salt
- Coconut flour, .5 c
- Grated coconut, .5 c
- Coconut milk, 2 c

What to Do

1. Place a saucepan on the stove on low heat. Pour in the coconut milk.
2. Whisk in the salt, nutmeg, cinnamon, flaxseed, and flour. Increase the heat and cook until it is just bubbling.
3. Add in the vanilla and continue to cook until as thick as you want it.
4. Spoon into bowls and top with blueberries.
5. Divide into four storage containers. Once completely cooled, place into refrigerator for five days.

Egg Cups with Hollandaise

This recipe makes 6 servings and contains 428 calories; 42 g fat; 9 g protein; 2 g net carbs per serving

What You Need

- EVOO, .25 c
- Cayenne
- Salt, .5 tsp.
- Zest and juice of a lemon
- Hot water, .5 c
- Halved avocado
- Pepper
- Eggs, 6
- Bacon, 6 slices

What to Do

1. Set your oven to 400.
2. Place the bacon in the bottom of six cups of a cupcake tin. Sprinkle in some pepper.
3. Let the bacon bake for ten minutes.
4. Take the bacon out of the oven and then carefully crack an egg into each c.
5. Place this back in the oven and let it cook for ten more minutes, or until the eggs are cooked to your desired doneness.
6. Meanwhile, add the cayenne, salt, lemon zest and juice, hot water, and avocado to a blender. Blend the mixture until it forms a smooth consistency. You may want to pause and scrape down the sides a time or two.
7. As the blender is running, drizzle in the oil until it is completely incorporated. Evenly divide the sauce between six storage containers.
8. Once the eggs have finished cooking, carefully take them out of the muffin tin.
9. Place an egg into six storage containers. When you are ready to serve, drizzle with the hollandaise sauce.

10. The hollandaise and egg cups need to be stored in separate containers in the fridge. The hollandaise will last a couple of days, so it is best to make it on demand. The eggs cups will last in the fridge for four days.

Asparagus Breakfast Muffins

This recipe makes 6 servings and contains 411 calories; 31 g fat; 27 g protein; 7 g net carbs per serving

What You Need

- Pepper
- Salt, .5 tsp.
- Rosemary, 1 tsp.
- Dijon, 1 tsp.
- Heavy cream, .25 c
- Beaten eggs, 10
- Shredded Swiss cheese, 1 c
- Trimmed asparagus cut into bite-sized chunks, 1 lb.
- Chopped onion, .5
- Chopped bacon, 8 oz.
- Unsalted butter, 4 tbsp.
- EVOO or coconut oil – for greasing

What to Do

1. Prepare a 12-c muffin tin and then grease them. Set to 375 degrees the temperature of your oven.
2. Add the butter to a large skillet and cook until it starts to bubble. Put in the bacon and cook until it has browned. This will take about five minutes.
3. Mix in the asparagus and onion. Stir occasionally. Cook until they become tender or for approximately five minutes
4. Spoon this into the muffin cups.
5. Sprinkle with cheese.
6. Mix together the pepper, salt, rosemary, mustard, cream, and eggs.
7. In the muffin cups, pour in the egg mixture.
8. Cook this in the oven for 12-15 minutes, or until the eggs are completely cooked through. Take these out and carefully take the muffins out of the tin. Using six storage containers, add two muffins. Allow them to cool completely before covering the containers.
9. This will keep in the fridge for three days or will freeze for up to six months. Place them in the fridge overnight to thaw and then microwave

for a couple of minutes. You can also slide them in the oven at 375 for ten minutes.

Tex-Mex Scramble

This recipe makes 4 servings and contains 508 calories; 40 g fat; 32 g protein; 5 g net carbs per serving

What You Need

- Shredded cheddar, .5 c
- Beaten eggs, 8
- Minced garlic, 2 cloves
- Minced jalapeno
- Chopped scallions, 6
- Bulk chorizo, 8 oz.

What to Do

1. Add the chorizo to a large skillet and cook until it has browned up. Make sure that you break the chorizo up as you go. This will take about five minutes.

2. Add in the jalapeno and scallions. Stir the mixture occasionally, until softened. This will take about an extra three minutes.

3. Mix in the garlic.

4. Add in the eggs.

5. Cook the mixture, scrambling the eggs as they cook through.

6. Sprinkle in the cheese. Stir everything together.

7. For meal prepping, divide the eggs between four containers.

8. This will keep in the refrigerator for three days, or you can freeze them up for six months. To thaw them out, let them rest in the fridge overnight and then microwave for a couple of minutes.

Egg Stuffed Peppers

This recipe makes 4 servings and contains 459 calories; 6 g net carbs per serving; 33 g protein; 34 g fat

What You Need

- Parmesan, .5 c
- Red pepper flakes
- Pepper
- Salt, .5 tsp.
- Italian seasoning, 1 tsp.
- Heavy cream, .25 c
- Beaten eggs, 8
- Sliced mushrooms, 4 oz.
- Bulk Italian sausage, .5 lb.

What to Do

1. Start by heating your oven to 400.
2. On a baking sheet, place the peppers with the cut-side up. Bake them for five minutes, or until they have softened up.
3. Meanwhile, add the sausage to a large skillet and cook until browned, breaking the meat up as it cooks. This will take about five minutes.
4. Mix in the mushrooms. Stir occasionally until the mushrooms become soft. This will take another five minutes. Let this cool slightly.
5. Beat the red pepper flakes, pepper, salt, Italian seasoning, cream, and eggs together.
6. Fold the cooled mushrooms and sausage into the egg mixture.
7. Divide this mixture between the pepper halves and top them with the cheese.
8. Place this back in the oven. Allow the peppers to cook until the eggs have set and the cheese on top has browned. This will take about 40 minutes. Allow the peppers to cool off before storing.
9. Place one stuffed pepper half in four containers.
10. These will keep for five days in the fridge or six months in the freezer. Thaw them in the refrigerator overnight and then microwave them for a

couple of minutes. You can also heat them up in the oven at 400 for 30 minutes.

Pancakes

This recipe makes 6 servings and contains 518 calories; 40 g fat; 13 g protein; 15 g net carbs per serving

What You Need

- Salt
- Baking soda, 2 tsp.
- Erythritol, 1 tbsp.
- Coconut flour, 1 c
- Vanilla, 1 tsp.
- Beaten eggs, 8
- Heavy cream, 1 c
- Melted butter, 1 c

What to Do

1. Whisk the vanilla, eggs, cream, and butter together.
2. Whisk the salt, baking soda, erythritol, and coconut flour together in a separate bowl.
3. In the coconut flour mixture, pour the egg mixture and stir together until it just comes together.
4. Brush some of the melted butter onto a heated skillet.
5. Cook a quarter of a c of the batter onto the pan until bubbles start to form on the top. This will take about two minutes.
6. Flip the pancake, and cook for a couple of minutes more.
7. Continue this process until you use up all of the pancake batter. It should make 18 pancakes.
8. Using six storage containers, place three pancakes into each.
9. These will keep for five days in the refrigerator and will keep in the freezer for six months. Let them thaw overnight in the refrigerator and heat in the microwave for a minute. You can also bake them at 350 for five to ten minutes.

Main Dishes

Keto Lasagna

This recipe makes 12 servings and contains 554 calories; 43 g fat; 29 g protein; 9 g net carbs per serving

What You Need

- Shredded mozzarella, 3 c – divided
- Sliced salami, 16 oz.
- Whole-milk ricotta, 16 oz.
- Pesto, 7 oz.
- Bulk Italian sausage, 1 lb.
- Italian seasoning, 1 tsp.
- Crushed tomatoes, 2 14-oz. cans – drain the juices off of one can
- Minced garlic, 6 cloves
- Minced shallot
- Avocado oil, .25 c

What to Do

1. Start by placing your oven to 350.

2. In a large skillet, heat the oil until it simmers.

3. Add in the shallow and let it cook for two minutes. Make sure you stir often. Cook in the garlic, stirring constantly, and until it smells delicious.

4. Mix in the tomatoes, as well as the juices of one can, and the Italian seasoning. Let this come up to a simmer. Let this cook, stirring occasionally, for five minutes.

5. Meanwhile, place the sausage in a large skillet and cook until browned. Make sure you break the sausage up as it cooks. This will take about five minutes. Take this off the heat and set to the side.

6. Mix together the ricotta and pesto.

7. Prepare a casserole dish with a 9"x13" size. In its bottom, pour in the sauce about one-half c.

8. Place a layer of salami over the sauce and then smooth over a layer of the ricotta mixture. Pour a dash of 1 c mozzarella on top. Add a quarter to a half of a c of the meat mixture over top. Place on another layer of salami and another layer of ricotta, and top with a c of mozzarella.

9. Place one last layer of salami over the top and cover with the rest of the sauce. Top with the rest of the mozzarella.

10. Place this on a rimmed baking sheet in case the lasagna boils over. Place this in the oven and let it bake for an hour. Let the lasagna cool slightly and then slice it into 12 pieces.

11. Place a square of lasagna into 12 storage containers.

12. The lasagna will keep refrigerated for five days or frozen for six months. Reheat the lasagna at 350 for 45 minutes.

Cabbage and Pork Stir-Fry

This recipe makes 6 servings and contains 698 calories; 4 g net carbs per serving; 54 g protein; 50 g fat

What You Need

- Chili oil, .5 tsp.
- Sesame oil, .5 tsp.
- Soy sauce, 1 tbsp.
- Juice of 2 limes
- Minced garlic, 3 cloves
- Freshly grated ginger, 1 tbsp.
- Shredded cabbage, 2 c
- Sliced scallions, 6
- Ground pork, 1 lb.
- Coconut oil, 3 tbsp.

What to Do

1. Pour the coconut oil to a large frying pan and let it heat up until it starts to shimmer.

2. Add in the pork and cook until it browns up. Break it apart as it cooks. This will take about five minutes.

3. Place the ginger, cabbage, and scallions. Stir constantly and cook until the vegetables have softened up. This will take about three minutes.

4. Cook the garlic next until they all smell delicious.

5. Mix in the chili oil, sesame oil, soy sauce, and lime juices. Cook the mixture for one to two minutes, or until everything is heated.

6. Divide the mixture between six containers.

7. This will keep in the refrigerator for three days or will last for six months in the freezer. Thaw them in the fridge overnight and microwave a couple of minutes to heat through.

Glazed Meatloaf

This recipe makes 6 servings and contains 265 calories; 15 g fat; 24 g protein; 2 g net carbs per serving

What You Need

- Pepper
- Salt
- Balsamic vinegar, 1 tbsp.
- Eggs, 2
- Parmesan cheese, .33 c
- Almond flour, .5 c
- Chopped mushrooms, 1 c
- Chopped parsley, 2 tbsp.
- Minced garlic, 4 cloves
- Chopped onion, 1
- Chopped bell pepper, 1
- Ground beef, 3 lbs.
- Glaze Ingredients:
- Stevia, 1 tbsp.
- Balsamic vinegar, 2 c
- Zero-sugar ketchup, .25 c

What to Do

1. You need to warm your oven to 375.
2. Place all the ingredients for the meatloaf into a large bowl. Hand-mix all of the ingredients so that they are combined thoroughly.
3. Place the mixture into a 13" x 9" casserole dish and shape into an oval loaf.
4. Put into the oven and bake for 30 minutes.
5. To make the glaze, put the stevia, balsamic vinegar, and ketchup into a small saucepan on medium heat. Stir until combined. Make sure it doesn't boil.
6. Carefully take out of the oven and spread the glaze on top.
7. Bake in the oven again for another twenty mins.
8. Carefully remove and let cool for a few minutes.

9. Slice any unused portion and place into storage containers. Place into the freezer for six months or in the fridge for five days.

Thai Beef

This recipe makes 6 servings and contains 226 calories; 19 g fat; 19 g protein; 2 g net carbs per serving

What You Need

- Pepper
- Salt
- Chopped green onion, 3
- Chopped bell pepper, 1
- Lemon pepper, 1.5 tsp.
- Beef broth, 1 c
- Peanut butter, 4 tbsp.
- Beefsteak, 1 pound
- Olive oil, 2 tbsp.
- Coconut aminos, 1 tbsp.
- Onion powder, .25 tsp.
- Garlic powder, .25 tsp.

What to Do

1. Into a bowl, add the lemon pepper, coconut aminos, beef broth, and peanut butter. Mix well to combine.

2. Slice up the steak into strips.

3. Put a large skillet onto the stove on medium and warm up two tablespoons of olive oil.

4. When heated, add in the steak, garlic powder, onion powder, pepper, and salt. Sauté for seven minutes.

5. Add in the bell pepper and cook for an additional three minutes.

6. Pour in the peanut butter mixture and onions. Cook for an additional two minutes, stirring frequently.

7. Using six storage containers, evenly divide. Store in the refrigerator for five days or freeze for six months.

Meatballs and Mushroom Sauce

This recipe makes 6 servings and contains 436 calories; 26 g fat; 32 g protein; 2 g net carbs per serving

What You Need

- Meatball Ingredients:
- Chopped parsley, 1 tbsp.
- Coconut flour, .75 c
- Beef broth, .25 c
- Coconut aminos, 1 tbsp.
- Garlic powder, 1 tsp.
- Pepper
- Salt
- Chopped jalapeno, 1
- Chopped onion, 1
- Ground beef, 2 lbs.
- Mushroom Sauce Ingredients:
- Pepper
- Salt
- Beef broth, .5 c
- Sour cream, .25 c
- Coconut aminos, 1 tsp.
- Chopped onions, 1 c
- Sliced mushrooms, 2 c
- Olive oil, 2 tbsp.
- Butter, 2 tbsp.

What to Do

1. You need to warm your oven to 375.
2. Take a baking sheet and line it with parchment paper.
3. In a large dish, place the entire meatball ingredients. Using your hands, mix until all ingredients are combined well.
4. Form into meatballs and place onto prepared baking sheet.
5. Put into the oven and bake 20 minutes.
6. Place a saucepan on medium heat and warm the olive oil.
7. When heated, add mushrooms and cook four minutes, stirring frequently.

8. Add onions and cook an additional four minutes.

9. Add in the beef stock, sour cream, and coconut aminos. Stir well to combine. Cook until everything is warmed through.

10. Take off heat and season with pepper and salt.

11. Take the meatballs out of the oven and drizzle mushroom sauce over the meatballs.

12. Divide evenly into storage containers and either place into the refrigerator for five days or freeze for six months.

Roasted Pork Belly

This recipe makes 6 servings and contains 367 calories; 2 g net carbs per serving; 31 g protein; 38 g fat

What You Need

- Cored and wedged apples, 3
- Pepper
- Salt
- Chopped parsley, 2 tbsp.
- Garlic, 4 cloves
- Chopped onion, 1
- Scored pork belly, 2 lbs.
- Stevia, 2 tbsp.
- Lemon juice, 1 tbsp.
- Olive oil, 3 tbsp.

What to Do

1. Put the apples, pepper, salt, parsley, garlic, onion, one c of water, lemon juice, and stevia into a blender. Process until almost smooth.

2. Place the pork belly into a steamer tray and steam for one hour. Take out of the steamer and set to the side.

3. You need to warm your oven to 425.

4. Take three tablespoons of olive oil and rub over pork. The apple mixture should be poured on top of the pork.

5. Put into a preheated oven for 30 minutes or until cooked through.

6. Allow to cool.

7. Slice the pork and divide into six containers place into the refrigerator for five days or freeze for six months.

Lamb Meatballs

This recipe makes 4 servings and contains 286 calories; 2 g net carbs per serving; 21 g protein; 24 g fat

What You Need

- Pepper
- Salt
- Paprika, .5 tsp.
- Shredded cheddar, .25 c
- Egg, 1
- Garlic powder, .5 tsp.
- Onion powder, .5 tsp.
- Coconut flour, .5 c
- Ground lamb, 1.5 lb.

What to Do

1. You need to warm your oven to 400.

2. Take a baking sheet and line it with parchment paper.

3. Place the pepper, salt, paprika, onion powder, garlic powder, egg, cheese, coconut flour, and lamb into a large bowl. Using your hands, mix until thoroughly combined.

4. Shape into meatballs and put onto the prepared baking sheet.

5. Put into the oven and bake for 15 minutes.

6. Divide evenly into storage containers and place into the refrigerator for five days or in the freezer for up to six months.

Mushroom Pork Chops

This recipe makes 4 servings and contains 599 calories; 4 g net carbs per serving; 30 g protein; 13 g fat

What You Need

- Pepper
- Salt
- Mayonnaise, 1 c
- Chopped onion, 1
- Minced garlic, 2 cloves
- Sliced mushrooms, 1.5 c
- Coconut oil, 4 tbsp.
- Balsamic vinegar, 1 tbsp.
- Pork chops, 4

What to Do

1. You need to warm your oven to 350.

2. Place a large skillet onto the stove on medium heat and melt two tablespoons coconut oil. Add in the onion, mushrooms, and garlic. Sauté for four minutes. Take off heat and set to the side.

3. Sprinkle the pork chops with pepper and salt.

4. Add the rest of the coconut oil to the skillet. When heated, add the pork chops and brown on each side.

5. Place into a baking dish and put into the oven. Bake for 30 minutes.

6. When done, remove the pork chops carefully and set to the side.

7. Place a saucepan on medium heat. Add in the mushroom mixture, mayonnaise, and balsamic vinegar. Stir until everything is combined. Take off heat.

8. Drizzle the sauce over pork.

9. Using four storage containers, add one pork chop to each. Store in the refrigerator for five days or freezer for six months.

Zesty Halibut

This recipe makes 4 servings and contains 581 calories; 4 g net carbs per serving; 38 g protein; 46 g fat

What You Need

- Pepper, .25
- Salt, .25
- Olive oil, 2 tbsp.
- Chopped onions, .25 c
- Lime juice, 2 tbsp.
- Avocados, 2
- Chopped cauliflower, 1 head
- Boneless halibut, 4 6-oz. fillets

What to Do

1. Pulse the cauliflower in a food processor until it resembles rice.

2. Add a tablespoon of oil to a skillet. Cook the rice until it has become tender or for about eight minutes. Take the rice out and set it to the side.

3. In a clean food processor, mix the onion, lime juice, and avocado until smooth.

4. Add the rest of the oil to the skillet.

5. Rub the fish with pepper and salt. You can also add on any other spices that you would like.

6. Place the fish in the skillet, working in batches if you need to, and cook four to five minutes on each side.

7. Once the fish is cooked through, place a fillet in four storage containers and divide the cauliflower rice between the four bowls. Divide the avocado sauce between four single-serving dressing cups. When ready to enjoy, drizzle the sauce over everything and serve.

8. This cannot be frozen. It will last five days in the refrigerator.

Bok Choy Stir-Fry

This recipe makes 4 servings and contains 68 calories; 1 g net carbs per serving; 3 g protein; 6 g fat

What You Need

- White pepper, .5 tsp.
- Fish sauce, 1 tsp.
- Sliced red bell pepper
- Sliced leeks, 2
- Minced garlic, 4 cloves
- Coconut oil, 2 tbsp.
- Coconut aminos, 2 tbsp.
- Sliced shitake mushrooms, 1 c
- Chopped bok choy, 4 c

What to Do

1. Add the coconut oil to a skillet and once heated, add in the mushrooms, bell pepper, garlic, and leeks. Cook the vegetables until they have softened up. Stir occasionally.

2. Add in the bok choy and cook for another four minutes. Stir occasionally.

3. Mix in the pepper, fish sauce, and coconut aminos. Let this cook for another minute.

4. Divide the stir-fry between four storage containers.

5. You can keep for five days in the refrigerator. You can also freeze it up to six months. To reheat, let it thaw overnight and then add it to a skillet to heat through.

Chicken Quesadilla

This recipe makes 4 servings and contains 599 calories; 41 g fat; 53 g protein; 8 g net carbs per serving

What You Need

- Pepper, .25 tsp.
- Salt, .5 tsp.
- Sliced avocados, 1
- Low-carb wraps, 4
- Grilled chicken breasts, 4
- Favorite shredded cheese, 1 c
- Minced jalapeno, 4 tsp.

What to Do

1. Place one of the low-carb wraps on the frying pan. Cook the wrap for two minutes on each side and then sprinkle a quarter c of the cheese over the wrap. Place a shredded chicken breast, a teaspoon of jalapeno, and some avocado slice to one have of the wrap.

2. Carefully fold the wrap over the chicken and flatten out.

3. Take the wrap out and continue with the other three wraps.

4. Place one wrap in a storage container.

5. This will keep for five days in the fridge and up to six months in the freezer. To reheat, let it thaw overnight in the refrigerator and then warm in the oven for ten minutes at 350.

Spinach and Artichoke Chicken

This recipe makes 4 servings and contains 450 calories; 2 g net carbs per serving; 39 g protein; 24 g fat

What You Need

- Pepper, .5 tsp.
- Chopped onion, .5
- Minced garlic, 2 cloves
- Salt, 1 tsp.
- Parmesan, .5 c
- Spinach, 2.5 c
- Chopped artichoke hearts, 2.5c
- Cream cheese, 4 oz.
- Shredded mozzarella, .5 c
- Boneless skinless chicken breasts,

What You Need

1. Start by placing your oven to 400.
2. Grease a casserole dish and rub the chicken pepper and salt.
3. After placing the chicken in the casserole dish, bake for thirty minutes.
4. As the chicken is cooking, mix together the garlic, cream cheese, parmesan, spinach, onions, and artichokes. Make sure the mixture is well combined.
5. When the 30 minutes are up, carefully take the casserole dish out of the oven. Slice a pocket in the middle of each of the chicken breasts.
6. Divide the artichoke mixture between the four chicken breasts, stuffing it inside of the pocket.
7. The shredded mozzarella should then be sprinkled over the chicken.
8. Bake it again in the oven for an additional fifteen minutes.
9. Check to make sure the chicken reached 165.
10. Once done, allow it to cool off before placing a chicken breast in a storage container.

11. This will keep in the refrigerator for five days. You can also freeze it for up to six months. To reheat, let it thaw in the refrigerator and then microwave it for a couple of minutes.

Chicken Soup

This recipe makes 4 servings and contains 381 calories; 3 g net carbs per serving; 31 g protein; 23 g fat

What You Need

- Chopped celery, .5 c
- Sour cream, .5 c
- Pepper, 1 tsp.
- Shredded chicken, 2 c
- Cream cheese, 4 oz.
- Butter, 3 tbsp.
- Salt, 1 tsp.
- Chicken stock, 4 c

What to Do

1. Add the sour cream, pepper, salt, butter, cream cheese, and chicken stock to a blender and mix until everything is well combined.

2. Pour this into a large pot. Add in the chicken, carrots, and celery.

3. Once the mixture boils, simmer it on low heat. Let it cook for a few minutes until everything has heated through.

4. Divide the soup between four bowls.

5. This will keep for five days in the refrigerator or you can freeze it for up to six months. When you want to reheat it, let the soup thaw in the refrigerator overnight and then add to a pot to heat it through.

Lamb Goulash

This recipe makes 6 servings and contains 287 calories; 3 g net carbs per serving; 11 g protein; 12 g fat

What You Need

- Ground lamb, 1.5 lbs.
- Cauliflower florets, 2 c
- Chicken broth, 1.5 cups
- Diced tomatoes, 1 14.5 oz. can
- Tomato paste, 1 tbsp.
- Chopped onion, 1
- Chopped red bell pepper, 1
- Chopped bell pepper, 1
- Water, 1.5 c
- Salt
- Pepper

What to Do

1. On medium heat, place a large pan. The ground lamb should be added next. Cook until no longer pink.

2. Add in the bell peppers and onion. Continue to cook for another four minutes, stirring frequently.

3. Add in the water, diced tomatoes, and cauliflower. Give everything a good stir and allow to simmer.

4. Place a lid on the skillet and cook for five minutes.

5. Add in seasonings and tomato paste and stir well to combine.

6. Take off heat and allow to cool. Cool completely and transfer to storage containers. Store in the refrigerator for five days or in the freezer for six months.

Mediterranean Pork

This recipe makes 4 servings and contains 241 calories; 1 g net carbs per serving; 28 g protein; 19 g fat

What You Need

- Pepper, 1 tsp.
- Salt, 1 tsp.
- Minced garlic, 4 cloves
- Greens of choice, 4 c
- Chopped zucchini
- Halved cherry tomatoes, 1 c
- Rosemary, 4 tsp.
- Olive oil, 4 tbsp.
- Bone-in pork chops, 4

What to Do

1. Start by placing your oven at 425.
2. Rub the pork chops with the oil, pepper, garlic, salt, and rosemary.
3. Place them on a baking sheet and slide into the oven. Let the pork chops bake for ten minutes.
4. Turn the heat down to 350 and let them continue to cook for 25 minutes. Remove the chops and let them cool off before storing.
5. Meanwhile, toss together the greens, zucchini, and tomatoes.
6. In four storage containers, divide out the salad mixture and add in one pork chop.
7. This will keep for five days in the refrigerator.

Slow Cooker Chili

This recipe makes 8 servings and contains 466 calories; 36 g fat; 31 g protein; 4 g net carbs per serving

What You Need

- Sour cream, 1 c
- Shredded cheddar, 1 c
- Salt, 1 tsp.
- Cumin, 1 tsp.
- Garlic powder, 1 tsp.
- Ground coriander, 1 tsp.
- Chili powder, 3 tbsp.
- Chopped onion
- Boneless pork shoulder cut into cubes, 2 lbs.

What You Need

1. Place everything except for the sour cream and cheese in your slow cooker and stir everything together.

2. Place the lid on the cooker and set it to low for eight hours or on high for four hours.

3. Once the chili is done, allow it to cool and add 1 ½ cups of chili into eight storage containers. When you are ready to serve, top with some sour cream and cheese.

4. This will keep for five days in the refrigerator or six months in the freezer. Allow the chili to thaw overnight in the fridge and then microwave for a couple of minutes. You can also reheat on the stovetop, stirring occasionally, until it has heated through. You can add in a little broth if the chili is too thick.

Slow Cooke Stew

This recipe makes 8 servings and contains 933 calories; 66 g fat; 69 g protein; 6 g net carbs per serving

What You Need

- Pepper, .25 tsp.
- Salt, 1 tsp.
- Rosemary, 1 tsp.
- Thyme, 1 tsp.
- Dijon, 1 tbsp.
- Garlic powder, 2 tsp.
- Dry red wine, 1 c
- Chopped celery, 4 stalks
- Bag frozen pearl onion, 8 oz.
- Halved or quartered button mushrooms, 1 lb.
- Chopped onions, 2
- Stew meat cut into cubes, 1 ½ lb.

What to Do

1. Add all of the ingredients to your slow cooker and stir everything together.

2. Place on the lid and set your cooker to low for eight hours or on high for four hours. Allow the stew to cool off.

3. Add 1 ½ cups of stew to eight storage containers.

4. The stew will last for five days in the refrigerator or for six months in the freezer. Allow this to thaw overnight in the refrigerator and then microwave for a couple of minutes. You can also heat it through on the stovetop. You can add in some broth if it is too thick.

Burrito Bowls

This recipe makes 4 servings and contains 528 calories; 35 g fat; 41 g protein; 12 g net carbs per serving

What You Need

- Chopped avocado
- Sour cream, .5 c
- Shredded cheddar, 1 c
- Cooked cauliflower rice, 2 c
- Sliced bell pepper
- Slice onion
- Pork belly, 1 lb.
- Minced scallions, 6
- Minced garlic, 6 cloves
- Salt, .5 tsp.
- Minced jalapeno
- Juice of 3 limes
- Chopped cilantro, 1 bunch
- Avocado oil, .5 c – divided

What You Need

1. Mix together the scallions, garlic, salt, jalapeno, lime juice, cilantro, and a quarter c of oil. Reserve two tablespoons of the mixture.

2. Add the rest of the mixture to a baggie and add in the pork belly. Shake it around so that the pork gets coated. Seal up the bag and allow it to be refrigerated for four to eight hours.

3. Heat up the remaining oil in a large skillet until it starts to shimmer.

4. Take the meat out of the marinade and wipe away the excess. Place the meat in the oil, cooking until it reaches 145. This will take about five minutes on each side. Place this on a plate and tent it with foil.

5. Using the same skillet, add in the bell pepper and onion. Occasionally stir the veggies. Cook for about five minutes, or until they become soft.

6. Thinly slice the meat against the grain and add it back into the pan. Mix in the reserved marinade. Cook the meat mixture for two more minutes, or until everything is coated with the marinade.

7. Divide the meat and veggies between four storage containers. In four other containers, add ½ c of the cauliflower rice. When you are ready to eat, mix the rice and meat mixture and top with the avocado, sour cream, and cheese.

8. These will keep for five days in the refrigerator. Reheat them for a couple of minutes in the microwave.

Chicken Casserole

This recipe makes 8 servings and contains 609 calories; 56 g fat; 25 g protein; 9 g net carbs per serving

What You Need

- Shredded cheddar, 1 c
- Cream of mushroom soup, 10.5 oz. can
- Bag frozen pearl onions, 8 oz.
- Halved button mushrooms, 1 lb.
- Bone-in chicken thighs, 8

What to Do

1. Start by setting your oven to 350.

2. Place the chicken thighs into the bottom of a 9" x 13" casserole dish. Add in the onions and mushrooms. Make sure that they are mixed up, but scattered across the pan.

3. Mix the cheese and soup together and pour the mixture over the chicken.

4. Cover the dish with aluminum foil and bake it for an hour and 15 minutes, or until the chicken has reached 165 and the juices run clear. Allow this to cool.

5. In eight storage containers, place a chicken thigh along with some of the vegetables and sauce.

6. This will keep for six months in the freezer and three days in the refrigerator. Allow it to thaw overnight in the fridge and then reheat it for a couple of minutes in the microwave. You can also bake it for 20-30 minutes at 375.

Tuna Casserole

This recipe makes 9 servings and contains 761 calories; 59 g fat; 53 g protein; 9 g net carbs per serving

What You Need

- Shredded cheddar, 1 c
- Oil-packed tuna, 1 lb. –drained
- Dijon, 1 tbsp.
- Dried dill, 1 tsp.
- Zest of a lemon
- Cream of mushroom soup, 10.5 oz. can
- Minced garlic, 3 cloves
- Sliced zucchini, 2
- Chopped onion
- Avocado oil, .25 c

What to Do

1. Start by placing your oven to 350.
2. Add the oil to a large skillet and heat it up until it shimmers. Add in the zucchini and onion, stirring occasionally, and cook until they start to soften up. This will take about five minutes.
3. Mix in the garlic and cook for about 30 seconds, or until it becomes fragrant. Take this off of the heat and let it cool.
4. Mix together the mustard, dill, lemon zest, and mushroom soup. Whisk it until smooth. Stir in the cooled veggies, cheese, and tuna. Stir well.
5. Spread this into a 9" x 13" casserole dish. Bake the casserole until it is bubbly, around an hour. Allow the casserole to cool.
6. Divide the casserole between nine storage containers.
7. This will keep for three days in the refrigerator and six months in the freezer. Let it thaw in the refrigerator overnight and microwave for a couple of minutes. You can also bake it for 15-20 minutes at 375.

Fettuccine Alfredo

This recipe makes 6 servings and contains 691 calories; 62 g fat; 29 g protein; 8 g net carbs per serving

What You Need

- Pepper
- Parmesan, 1 c
- Heavy cream, .5 c
- Butter, 8 tbsp.
- Cream cheese, 8 oz.
- Minced garlic, 3 cloves
- Spiralized zucchini, 4
- Sliced mushrooms, 8 oz.
- Minced shallot, 2 tbsp.
- Cubed pancetta, 6 oz.
- EVOO, 4 tbsp. – divided

What to Do

1. Add two tablespoons of oil into a large skillet and let it heat up until it shimmers. Add in the pancetta and cook it until it has browned up. This will take about five minutes. With a slotted spoon, remove the pancetta and set it to the side.

2. Add in the rest of the oil and cook the mushrooms and shallot. Stir occasionally until they have browned up. This will take about five minutes. Mix in the zucchini and cook for three minutes more. The zucchini should become tender. Add in the garlic and cook until the garlic becomes fragrant. Make sure you stir constantly. Mix the pancetta back in and cook for another 30 seconds to warm the pancetta back up.

3. As the veggies are cooking, add the pepper, parmesan, cream, butter, and cream cheese to a pot. Heat and stir until everything has melted together. Whisk everything until they are heated through, about five minutes.

4. Divide the veggies between four containers, placing them to one side. Divide the sauce in the same containers, placing it on the other side. When ready to eat, mix the sauce and veggies together.

5. This will keep for four days in the refrigerator and six months in the freezer. Let it thaw overnight in the fridge. Place everything in a pot and heat everything together until warm. You may need to add in some cream to adjust the consistency.

Arroz Con Pollo

This recipe makes 4 servings and contains 513 calories; 35 g fat; 31 g protein; 13 g net carbs per serving

What You Need

- Sour cream, .5 c
- Shredded Monterey Jack, 1 c
- Uncooked cauliflower rice, 2 c
- Cayenne
- Salt, .5 tsp.
- Garlic powder, 1 tsp.
- Cumin, 1 tsp.
- Oregano, 1 tsp.
- Chili powder, 1 tbsp.
- Crushed tomatoes, 14 oz.
- Sliced mushrooms, 8 oz.
- Chopped onion
- Chopped boneless skinless chicken thighs, 1 lb.
- Avocado oil, .25 c

What to Do

1. Add the oil to a large skillet and heat it up until it shimmers.

2. Add in the chicken and cook them, stirring occasionally, until it has browned. This will take about five minutes. With a slotted spoon, take the chicken out and set it to the side.

3. Mix in the mushrooms and onion. Stir occasionally, until the veggies have browned up. This will take about five minutes.

4. Place the chicken back in the skillet, along with any juices that may have collected.

5. Mix in the cayenne, salt, garlic powder, cumin, oregano, chili powder, and the can of tomatoes with their juices. Stir everything together and allow it to come to a simmer.

6. Mix in the cauliflower and cook for five minutes, stirring occasionally.

7. Mix in the cheese, stirring until the cheese is melted and incorporated.

8. Divide the mixture between four containers. Serve with a garnish of sour cream.

9. This will keep for five days in the fridge or for six months in the freezer. Allow it to thaw in the refrigerator overnight and then microwave it for a few minutes.

Chopped Chicken Salad

This recipe makes 4 servings and contains 499 calories; 40 g fat; 22 g protein; 12 g net carbs per serving

What You Need

- Red pepper flakes
- Pepper
- Salt, .5 tsp.
- Minced shallot, 1 tbsp.
- Apple cider vinegar, 3 tbsp.
- EVOO, .5 c
- Dijon, 2 tbsp.
- Quartered cherry tomatoes, 8
- Chopped and drained artichoke hearts, 14 oz. can
- Chopped red bell pepper
- Sliced black olives, .5 c
- Chopped hard-boil eggs, 2
- Chopped meat from a rotisserie chicken, 1 lb.

What to Do

1. Mix together the cherry tomatoes, artichoke hearts, bell pepper, olives, eggs, and chicken in a large bowl.

2. Mix together the red pepper flakes, pepper, salt, shallot, vinegar, oil, and mustard.

3. Place the chicken salad equally into four storage containers. Divide the vinaigrette between four single-serving dressing containers. Toss the salad in the dressing to serve.

4. This won't freeze, but it will keep for a week in the refrigerator.

Simple Salmon Salad

This recipe makes 4 servings and contains 446 calories; 31 g fat; 34 g protein; 9 g net carbs per serving

What You Need

- Pepper
- Dried dill, 1 tsp.
- Zest and juice of a lemon
- Dijon, 1 tsp.
- EVOO, 3 tbsp.
- Mayonnaise, .5 c
- Chopped dill pickles, 3
- Chopped scallions, 3
- Flaked salmon, 8 oz. can

What to Do

1. Mix together the pickles, scallions, and salmon.

2. Beat together the pepper, dill, lemon zest and juice, mustard, oil, and mayonnaise.

3. Mix the salmon and the dressing together.

4. Divide the mixture between four storage containers.

5. This won't freeze, but you can keep it stored for five days in the refrigerator.

Gyro Salad with Tzatziki

This recipe makes 3 servings and contains 501 calories; 31 g fat; 47 g protein; 10 g net carbs per serving

What You Need

- Pepper, .5 tsp.
- Salt, .5 tsp.
- Chopped dill, 1 tsp.
- Chopped mint, 2 tsp.
- Ripe avocado
- Thyme, .5 tsp.
- Oregano, .5 tsp.
- Juice of a lemon – divided
- Low-sodium chicken broth, .25 c
- Grated cucumber, 1 medium
- Chopped onion, .5
- Olive oil, 1 tbsp.
- Ground lamb meat, 1 lb.
- Chopped romaine, 6 c

What to Do

1. Heat the oil in a large skillet. Once the oil has become hot, add in the lamb and cook for three minutes.

2. Mix in the onion. Cook until the onion has become soft.

3. Mix in the thyme, oregano, lemon juice, and chicken broth. Season with the pepper and salt. Turn the heat up and allow it to simmer for five minutes.

4. Spread the grated cucumber out on a cheesecloth and squeeze as much liquid off of the cucumber as you can.

5. For the sauce, add the dill, mint, lemon juice, avocado, and cucumber to a food processor. Mix everything together until it becomes smooth.

6. Place the lettuce in three storage containers. Divide the lamb mixture between the same containers, making sure it stays to one side. Divide that sauce between three single-serving dressing containers. When you are ready to eat, pour the sauce over the meat and lettuce and toss together.

7. This should not be frozen unless you are storing the lamb mixture by itself. The lamb mixture will last five days in the refrigerator and they can be frozen by itself for up to six months. The tzatziki sauce will last for a week in the refrigerator.

Pepperoni Pizza

This recipe makes 6 servings and contains 563 calories; 44 g fat; 33 g protein; 5 g net carbs per serving

What You Need

- Pepper, .25 tsp.
- Salt, .5 tsp.
- Italian seasoning, 2 tsp.
- Chopped basil, 3 tbsp.
- Pepperoni slices, 2 oz. – divided
- Shredded mozzarella, .5 c – divided
- Low-carb tomato sauce, .66 c – divided
- EVOO, 3 tbsp.
- Psyllium husk powder, .25 c
- Grated parmesan, 8 tbsp.
- Eggs, 6

What to Do

1. Add the Italian seasoning, psyllium powder, parmesan, and eggs in a blender.
2. Blend the mixture together until smooth and then let it rest for five minutes.
3. Add a tablespoon of oil to a skillet.
4. Add in a third of the batter to the skillet. Cook the batter on both sides to create the crust. Do this twice more to use up the batter.
5. Place the crusts on a baking sheet and divide the tomato sauce over each crust.
6. Evenly divide the mozzarella and pepperoni on the crusts. Slide this under a broiler and cook until the cheese has melted and turned brown.
7. Sprinkle the top with some pepper, salt, and basil.
8. Allow the pizzas to cool off. Slice them each in half and place a half of a pizza into a storage container.
9. This will keep for five days in the refrigerator. This does not freeze well. To reheat, warm in the oven at 350 for ten minutes.

Double the Meat Stromboli

This recipe makes 6 servings and contains 533 calories; 38 g fat; 33 g protein; 7 g net carbs per serving

What You Need

- Pepper, .5 tsp.
- Salt, .5 tsp.
- Italian seasoning, 2 tsp.
- Coconut flour, .5 c
- Almond flour, .5 c
- Melted butter, 2 tbsp.
- Sliced cheddar, 1 c
- Sliced pepperoni, 4 oz.
- Sliced ham, 1 c
- Eggs, 2
- Shredded mozzarella, 2.5 c
- Salad greens, 12 c

What to Do

1. Start by placing your oven to 400.
2. Place parchment on a baking sheet.
3. Add the mozzarella to a microwave-safe bowl. Heat in 30-second increments until the cheese has melted, stirring each time until it becomes smooth.
4. Mix together the Italian seasoning, coconut flour, and almond flour.
5. Add in the melted cheese with the pepper and salt. Mix until everything has come together.
6. Stir in the eggs until the batter turns into dough.
7. Place this on the baking sheet. Lay another piece of parchment over top and use a rolling pin to roll the dough out into an oval shape.
8. Slice diagonal lines along the edges. Make sure that the middle four inches are not cut.
9. Layer the cheese, ham, and pepperoni in the middle of the dough. Fold the dough strips up over the toppings.

10. Brush the dough with some melted butter.

11. Slide the Stromboli into the oven and let it bake for 15-20 minutes or until it turns brown.

12. Slice the Stromboli into six equal sections.

13. Place a section into six containers. When you are ready to eat, serve with two cups of fresh salad greens.

14. I do not suggest freezing the Stromboli. It will keep in the fridge for five days.

Avocado Egg Salad

This recipe makes 6 servings and contains 348 calories; 28 g fat; 15 g protein; 4 g net carbs per serving

What You Need

- Pepper
- Salt
- Chopped red bell pepper, .5 pepper
- Chopped onion, .25
- Sliced avocados, 2
- Chopped hard-boiled eggs, 12

What to Do

1. Add the pepper, salt, bell pepper, onion, avocados, and eggs to a large bowl. Gently mix everything together until it is well-combined.

2. Divide the mixture between six storage containers.

3. This doesn't freeze well, but it will keep for five days in the refrigerator.

Herbed Turkey

This recipe makes 14 servings and contains 910 calories; 33 g fat; 47 g protein; 142 g net carbs per serving

What You Need

- Pepper, 1 tbsp.
- Salt, 1 tbsp.
- Whole garlic, 6 cloves
- Celery, 6 stalks
- Lemon, .5
- Large onion
- Thawed turkey, 15 lb.
- Coconut oil, 3 tbsp.
- Herbed Butter:
- Chopped parsley, .25 c
- Rosemary, 1 tbsp.
- Minced garlic, 4 cloves
- Butter, .5 c

What to Do

1. Place the herbed butter ingredients in a bowl and mix everything together. Set to the side but do not refrigerate.

2. Set your oven to 325.

3. Clean out the turkey cavities and rinse it with cold water until it runs clear. Pat the turkey dry.

4. Set the turkey in a large roasting pan that has been fitted with a roasting rack.

5. Place the celery, onion, garlic, and lemon wedges inside of the turkey.

6. Rub the turkey with the herbed butter and then drizzle the coconut oil over the top of the turkey.

7. Slide the turkey in the oven.

8. The turkey needs to cook for at least 20 minutes per pound. This will be around five hours. Check the temperature during the last few hours because it could get done early and you don't want the turkey to dry out. It needs to reach 165.

9. Remove the cooked turkey and allow it to rest for at least ten minutes before you carve.

10. If you are meal prepping, separate the carved meat equally between 14 storage containers.

11. This can be frozen for up to six months. When you reheat, you can use some more herbed butter to add moisture and flavor.

Tilapia with Avocado Salad

This recipe makes 8 servings and contains 382 calories; 23 g fat; 37 g protein; 6 g net carbs per serving

What You Need

- Halved cherry tomatoes, 1 c
- Diced avocado, 1 c
- Oregano, 1 tsp.
- Lemon zest, 2 tbsp.
- Lemon juice, 4 tbsp.
- Pepper, .5 tsp.
- Salt, .5 tsp.
- Minced garlic, 2 cloves
- Greek yogurt, 2 tbsp.
- Coconut oil, 5 tbsp.
- Tilapia fillets, 8 6-oz. fillets

What to Do

1. Mix together the pepper, salt, garlic, yogurt, lemon zest, and lemon juice. Stir in the coconut oil until everything comes together.
2. Place the tilapia in a bowl or a bag and cover with the yogurt mixture. Make sure that the fish is very well-coated.
3. Allow the fish to sit in the fridge for 20 minutes or overnight.
4. Set your oven to 400.
5. Lay the fish in a baking dish and slide it into the oven.
6. Bake the fish for 10-12 minutes. The fillets should easily flake with a fork.
7. Mix together a tablespoon of coconut oil with the tomatoes and avocados.
8. Using eight containers, place a tilapia fillet and a half of a c of the salad.
9. This will keep for five days in the refrigerator. I do not suggest freezing. Reheat the fish by itself in the microwave for a couple of minutes.

Fish Tacos

This recipe makes 4 servings and contains 301 calories; 21 g fat; 25 g protein; 2 g net carbs per serving

What You Need

- Large lettuce leaves, 4
- Minced chipotle peppers in adobo, 2
- Sliced jalapeno
- Chopped onion
- Olive oil, 2 tbsp.
- Butter, 2 tbsp.
- Mayonnaise, 2 tbsp.
- Coconut oil, 2 tbsp.
- Crushed garlic, 2 cloves
- Tilapia, 1 lb.

What to Do

1. Add two tablespoons of coconut oil to a skillet.
2. Once hot, add the onions and let them cook for about five minutes, or until they become translucent.
3. Turn the heat down and then mix in the garlic and jalapeno. Cook this for another two minutes, stirring occasionally. A word of advice, don't let your face be directly over the pan when you add the jalapeno. The fumes from the pepper will burn your eyes and throat.
4. Mince up the chipotle and mix them into the other vegetables.
5. Place the fish fillets in the skillet with the butter and mayonnaise.
6. Mix everything together and let it all cook together for eight minutes, or until the fish is cooked through.
7. To make your tacos, divide the fish mixture between the lettuce leaves.
8. For meal prep, divide the fish mixture between four containers. When ready to eat, heat the fish and wrap in a lettuce leaf.
9. This will keep for five days in the refrigerator. Do not freeze this dish.

Herbed Salmon

This recipe makes 4 servings and contains 211 calories; 12 g fat; 22 g protein; 1 g net carbs per serving

What You Need

- Sliced lemon, 2
- Onion powder, .5 tsp.
- Pepper, .5 tsp.
- Salt, .5 tsp.
- Olive oil, 2 tbsp.
- Whole garlic, 4 cloves
- Rosemary, 4 springs
- Chopped thyme, 1 tbsp.
- Chopped basil, 1 tbsp.
- Chopped parsley, 1 tbsp.
- Boneless salmon, 4 6-oz. fillets

What to Do

1. Start by placing your oven to 400.
2. Mix together the onion powder, pepper, salt, olive oil, thyme, basil, and parsley. Make sure it is very well-combined.
3. Place foil on a baking sheet and spray with cooking spray. Lay the salmon fillets on the baking sheet.
4. Rub the herbed mixture into the fish and top the salmon with lemon slices, a whole garlic clove, and a sprig of rosemary.
5. Slide this into the oven for 10-13 minutes. The salmon should flake easily with a fork.
6. For meal prep, place a salmon fillet in a storage container.
7. This should not be frozen, but it will keep in the fridge for five days.

Coconut Shrimp Soup

This recipe makes 4 servings and contains 289 calories; 26 g fat; 13 g protein; 3 g net carbs per serving

What You Need

- Pepper, .5 tsp.
- Salt, .5 tsp.
- Chopped cilantro, 2 tbsp.
- Grated ginger, 1 tsp.
- Basil, 1 tbsp.
- Fish sauce, 1 tbsp.
- Fish stock, 3 c
- Minced garlic, 4 cloves
- Chopped onion
- Melted coconut oil, 1 tbsp.
- Thai coconut milk, 14 oz. can
- Lime juice, 1 tbsp.
- Cleaned shrimp, 1 lb.

What to Do

1. Add the coconut oil to a large pot. Add in the garlic and onion. Cook for about six minutes, or until they have softened. Stir occasionally and don't let the garlic burn.

2. Add in the shrimp, cook, stirring occasionally until the shrimp turn pink.

3. Gently mix in all of the other ingredients and bring everything to a boil.

4. Once it has started to boil, lower the heat, and let it cook for 15 minutes at a simmer. Stir occasionally. Taste and adjust any of the seasonings that you need to.

5. Divide soup between four containers.

6. This can be kept for five months in the refrigerator. You can also store it in the freezer for six months. Let the soup thaw out in the fridge and reheat it in a pot until warmed through.

Crab Cakes

This recipe makes 4 servings and contains 303 calories; 18 g fat; 16 g protein; 3 g net carbs per serving

What You Need

- Chopped parsley, 1 tbsp.
- Paprika, .25 tsp.
- Garlic powder, .25 tsp.
- Onion powder, .25 tsp.
- Pepper, .5 tsp.
- Salt, .5 tsp.
- Mayonnaise, .25 c
- Dijon, 1 tsp.
- Butter, 4 tbsp.
- Coconut flour, 1 c
- Lump crab meat, 1.5 lb.

What You Need

1. Mix together the parsley, paprika, garlic powder, onion powder, pepper, salt, Dijon, and mayonnaise together.

2. Mix in the crab meat and make sure that everything is well combined and the crab is completely coated.

3. Slowly mix in the flour and stir everything together with your hands. Form the mixture into four patties.

4. Add the butter to a skillet, and once heated, place the crab cake in the pan and cook for four to six minutes on each side. Repeat this until all of the patties are cooked.

5. Place a crab cake into individual containers.

6. This cannot be frozen. This can be kept refrigerated for five days.

Specialty, Dessert, and Snacks

Almond Joy Fat Bomb

This recipe makes 12 servings and contains 188 calories; 21 g fat; <1 g protein; 2 g net carbs per serving

What You Need

- Liquid stevia
- Coconut oil, 1 c
- Unsweetened baking chocolate, 2 oz.
- Almond butter, 1 c

What to Do

1. Mix all of the ingredients together in a pot. Cook and stir the mixture until everything has melted and mixed together. Taste and add extra stevia if you need to.

2. Pour this mixture into mini muffin tins, ice cube trays, or candy molds.

3. Chill the fat bombs for at least an hour. Remove the fat bombs from their molds and keep in a storage container.

4. These will last for five days in the refrigerator or for six months in the freezer.

Strawberry Ice Pops

This recipe makes 4 servings and contains 272 calories; 27 g fat; 3 g protein; 6 g net carbs per serving

What You Need

- Liquid stevia, .5 tsp.
- Full-fat coconut milk, 13.6 oz. can
- Halved strawberries, 1 c

What to Do

1. Combine all of the ingredients together in a food processor or blender. Mix until the mixture becomes smooth.

2. Pour the mixture into ice pop molds and allow them to freeze overnight before you serve them.

3. This will keep in the freezer for six months.

Coconut Mousse

This recipe makes 6 servings and contains 396 calories; 41 g fat; 5 g protein; 6 g net carbs per serving

What You Need

- Vanilla, .5 tsp.
- Liquid stevia, 1 tsp.
- Espresso powder, 1 tsp.
- Melted and cooled unsweetened baking chocolate, 2 oz.
- Coconut milk, 2 13.6-oz. cans – use only the cream but reserve some of the milk if needed to reach your desired consistency

What to Do

1. Whisk all of the ingredients together until they are well combined. Use some of the coconut water if you need to thin out the mousse a little bit.

2. Divide the mouse between six containers.

3. This can keep for five days in the refrigerator. You can also freeze the mixture and slice into six squares to make fudge.

Stuffed Mushrooms

This recipe makes 8 servings and contains 162 calories; 13 g fat; 9 g protein; 4 g net carbs per serving

What You Need

- Stemmed button mushrooms, 1 lb.
- Parmesan, .5 c
- Minced shallot, 1 tbsp.
- Garlic powder, 1 tsp.
- Tabasco, 2 dashes
- Dijon, 1 tsp.
- Chopped frozen spinach, 4 oz. – thawed and wrung dry
- Room temperature cream cheese, 8 oz.

What to Do

1. Start by placing your oven to 425.
2. Mix together the parmesan, shallot, garlic powder, Tabasco, mustard, spinach, and cream cheese.
3. Lay the mushrooms in a baking sheet with the cap-side down.
4. Spoon a generous amount of the filling into each of the mushroom caps.
5. Allow this to bake for 25 minutes. Allow the mushrooms to cool off.
6. Divide the mushrooms into eight storage containers.
7. These won't freeze, but they keep in the refrigerator for five days. You can reheat in the microwave for a couple of minutes or for 25 minutes in an oven at 350.

Onion Dip with Crudités

This recipe makes 6 servings and contains 211 calories; 18 g fat; 4 g protein; 8 g net carbs per serving

What You Need

- Sliced bell peppers, 2
- Dijon, 1 tsp.
- Mayonnaise, .25 c
- Room temperature cream cheese, 8 oz.
- Salt, .5 tsp.
- Thyme, 1 tsp.
- Thinly sliced onions, 2
- Avocado oil, .25 c

What to Do

1. Add the oil to a skillet and heat until the oil begins to shimmer.

2. Turn the heat down and then add in the salt, thyme, and onions.

3. Cook the onions, stirring occasionally, until they have caramelized. This will take 20-30 minutes. Allow the onions to cool off.

4. Add the mustard, mayonnaise, cream cheese, and onions to a bowl and mix everything together. Make sure that everything is evenly distributed.

5. Using six storage containers, add a quarter c of dip. In six more storage containers, divide out the pepper strips. Even the pepper strips dipped into the onion dip.

6. The dip won't freeze, but it will all last about three days in the refrigerator.

Jalapeno Poppers

This recipe makes 8 servings and contains 240 calories; 20 g fat; 12 g protein; 3 g net carbs per serving

What You Need

- Crumbled cooked bacon, 8 slices
- Jalapeno peppers cut lengthwise with the ribs and seeds removed, 16
- Shredded pepper jack cheese, .5c
- Room temperature cream cheese, 6 oz.

What to Do

1. Start by placing your oven to 350.
2. Mix together the pepper jack cheese and the cream cheese until smooth.
3. Spoon this into the jalapeno halves and then lay them, with the cheese up, on a baking sheet. Sprinkle the bacon over the top of the cheese.
4. Bake the jalapeno poppers for 25 minutes, or until the cheese has melted and is bubbly.
5. Place four cooled poppers in eight storage containers.
6. These will keep in the fridge for five days. They don't freeze well. You can heat them up for two minutes in the microwave or 15-20 minutes at 350 in the oven.

Deviled Eggs

This recipe makes 6 servings and contains 72 calories; 6 g fat; 3 g protein; 3 g net carbs per serving

What You Need

- Salt, .5 tsp.
- Minced garlic, 1 clove
- Cayenne
- Minced scallions, 2
- Minced dill pickle
- Dijon, 1 tsp.
- Mayonnaise, .5 c
- Halved hard-boiled eggs, 6

What to Do

1. Remove the yolks from the whites and place them in a bowl. Lay the whites on a plate with the cut side up.

2. Mix together the salt, garlic, cayenne, scallions, pickle, mustard, mayonnaise, and yolks. Use a fork so that you can mash up the yolks as you go. Mix until they are well combined.

3. Place the yolk mixture into the egg whites either with a spoon or a piping bag.

4. Place two deviled eggs into six storage containers.

5. These will last for five days in the refrigerator.

Green Bean Casserole

This recipe makes 4 servings and contains 366 calories; 31 g fat; 15 g protein; 12 g net carbs per serving

What You Need

- Shredded cheddar, .5 c
- Caramelized onions, .5 c
- Cream of mushroom soup, 10.5 oz. can
- Cooked green beans, 3 c

What to Do

1. Start by placing your oven to 350.
2. Mix together all of the ingredients in a large bowl.
3. Spread the green bean mixture into the bottom of a 9" x 13" casserole dish. Bake the casserole for 15 minutes, or until it is hot and bubbly.
4. Allow the casserole to cool before you place it into storage containers.
5. Add a c of the casserole to four storage containers.
6. This will keep in the refrigerator for five days. It doesn't freeze well. To heat it up, bake it for 15 minutes at 350, or microwave it for a couple of minutes.

Roasted Brussels Sprouts

This recipe makes 4 servings and contains 347 calories; 26 g fat; 16 g protein; 10 g net carbs per serving

What You Need

- Pepper
- Salt, .5 tsp.
- Chopped bacon, 4 oz.
- Halved Brussels sprouts, 1.5 lbs.
- Avocado oil, .25 c

What to Do

1. Start by placing your oven to 400.

2. Toss together the pepper, salt, bacon, sprouts, and oil together so that the sprouts are well coated.

3. Lay the sprouts out on a baking sheet and bake them for 20 minutes. Flip the sprouts over halfway through the cooking time. You want them to brown up on both sides.

4. Once cooled, divide between four storage containers.

5. These will keep for five days in the refrigerator. You can freeze them, but the texture will become mushy once you reheat.

Mashed Cauliflower

This recipe makes 4 servings and contains 143 calories; 14 g fat; 3 g protein; 3 g net carbs per serving

What You Need

- Pepper
- Salt, .5 tsp.
- Heavy cream, .25 c
- Melted butter, .25 c
- Head of cauliflower

What to Do

1. Break apart the head of cauliflower into florets and place them in a pot of water and cover with water. Bring this to a boil.

2. Allow the cauliflower to boil for ten minutes, or until the cauliflower is soft.

3. Drain off the water. Place the cauliflower in a bowl and mash with a potato masher. Mix in the pepper, salt, cream, and butter. Mix until everything is incorporated and smooth.

4. Divide the mashed cauliflower between four containers.

5. You can keep in the refrigerator for five days or freeze it up to six months. Thaw it in the refrigerator overnight and then microwave for a couple of minutes to heat through. You can also heat it up on the stovetop. You may want to add a bit of cream to adjust the consistency.

Chopped Caprese Salad

This recipe makes 4 servings and contains 373 calories; 28 g fat; 25 g protein; 6 g net carbs per serving

What You Need

- Pepper
- Salt, .5 tsp.
- EVOO, .25 c
- Chopped mozzarella, 12 oz.
- Chopped basil leaves, 1 bunch
- Chopped heirloom tomatoes, 3 large

What to Do

1. Toss all of the ingredients together in a large bowl. Divide the salad between four containers.

2. Do not freeze this. It will keep, refrigerated, for three days.

Coleslaw

This recipe makes 4 servings and contains 103 calories; 7 g fat; 2 g protein; 7 g net carbs per serving

What You Need

- Salt, .5 tsp.
- Grated ginger, 1 tsp.
- Minced garlic clove
- Sesame seeds, 1 tbsp.
- Chinese hot mustard, .5 tsp.
- Sriracha, .5 tsp.
- Juice of a lime
- Avocado oil, .5 c
- Apple cider vinegar, .25 c
- Chopped cilantro, 1 bunch
- Chopped scallions, 6
- Shredded cabbage, 4 c

What to Do

1. Toss together the cilantro, scallions, and cabbage.

2. Whisk together the salt, ginger, garlic, sesame seeds, mustard, sriracha, lime juice, oil, and vinegar.

3. Add a c of the cabbage mixture to four storage containers. Using four single-serving dressing containers, add three tablespoons of the dressing. When you are ready to serve, toss the cabbage in the dressing.

4. Do not freeze this. The dressing will keep for a week in the fridge and the slaw will last five days.

Fat Bomb Vanilla Smoothie

This recipe makes 4 servings and contains 551 calories; 48 g fat; 28 g protein; 6 g net carbs per serving

What You Need

- Vanilla, 1 tsp.
- Powdered erythritol, 2 tbsp.
- Coconut oil, 3 tbsp.
- Ice cubes, 8
- Vanilla almond milk, .5 c
- Whipped cream, .5 c
- Heavy cream, 1 c
- Vanilla protein powder, 2 scoops

What to Do

1. Add all of the ingredients to your blender except for the whipped cream.

2. Blend the ingredients together for a minute, or until they become smooth.

3. Pour the mixture into four glass and top with the whipped cream.

4. If you are meal prepping, pour the smoothie mixture into cupcake tins. Freeze the mixture and pop a few out when you want a smoothie. Blend them together and enjoy.

Homemade Nutella

This recipe makes 24 servings and contains 173 calories; 33 g fat; 3 g protein; 2 g net carbs per serving

What You Need

- Salt, .25 tsp.
- Stevia, .5 c
- Vanilla, 1 tsp.
- Unsweetened coconut milk, .5 c
- Heavy cream, .5 c
- Coconut oil, 4 tbsp.
- Unsweetened cacao powder, .5 c
- Hazelnuts, 4 c

What to Do

1. Start by placing your oven to 325.
2. Place the hazelnuts on a cookie sheet and slide them in the oven. Roast the nuts for 10-15 minutes or until they have browned up.
3. Place the hazelnuts on a wet towel and rub them until the dark skin has come off.
4. Add the hazelnuts and all of the other ingredients to a blender and mix until it forms a smooth mixture.
5. Keep this stored in a mason jar.
6. Keep this in the refrigerator and will likely last a month if it doesn't get eaten faster. Spread two tablespoons on some berries, or add to a smoothie.

Peanut Butter Cookies

This recipe makes 15 servings and contains 107 calories; 10 g fat; 5 g protein; 2 g net carbs per serving

What You Need

- Salt
- Erythritol, .5 c
- Egg
- Peanut butter, 1 c

What to Do

1. Start by setting your oven to 350.

2. Place parchment paper on a baking sheet.

3. Stir together all of the ingredients until they are well combined.

4. Form 15 1-inch balls of cookie dough and place them on the baking sheet.

5. Press them down a bit with a fork and slide them into the oven.

6. Let the cookies bake for 10-15 minutes, or until the edges have browned up. If you like crispy cookies, cook for a bit longer. If you like soft cookies, don't cook them quite as long.

7. These will keep at room temp for a week. You can also freeze them for up to six months. Allow them to come to room temperature before eating.

Cloud Bread

This recipe makes 10 servings and contains 50 calories; 6 g fat; 3 g protein; 0 g net carbs per serving

What You Need

- Softened cream cheese, 3 oz.
- Cream of tartar, .25 tsp.
- Separated eggs, 3

What to Do

1. Start by placing your oven to 300.
2. Place parchment on a baking sheet.
3. Separate the eggs, placing the yolks and whites in separate bowls.
4. Add the cream of tartar to the egg whites and whip until they are fluffy and shiny.
5. Beat the cream cheese into the yolks until well mixed. Carefully fold the fluffy whites into the yolks.
6. Spoon out ten circles of the batter onto the baking sheet. Make sure that you keep them two inches apart so that they don't run into each other.
7. Slide these into the oven and bake them for 30 minutes or until they are browned and firm.
8. Keep these stored in the refrigerator. Do not freeze them. This will cause the bread to fall.

Parfait

This recipe makes 4 servings and contains 353 calories; 23 g fat; 22 g protein; 5 g net carbs per serving

What You Need

- Toasted flaxseeds, 1 c
- Sliced bananas, 4 medium
- Blueberries, 2 c
- Sliced strawberries, 2 c
- Full-fat yogurt, 4 c
- Desiccated coconut, 1 c
- Chopped macadamia nuts, 1 c
- Chopped toasted walnuts, 1.5 c

What to Do

1. With four mason jars, add a half c of yogurt into the bottom of each.
2. Layer the flaxseeds, bananas, blueberries, strawberries, coconut, macadamia nuts, and walnuts into each of the jars.
3. Top each with another half c of yogurt.
4. Keep these stored in the refrigerator for three days.

Peanut Butter Chocolate Chip Cookies

This recipe makes 16 servings and contains 215 calories; 13 g fat; 6 g protein; 2 g net carbs per serving

What You Need

- Sea salt
- Vanilla, 1 tsp.
- Cinnamon, 1 tbsp.
- Baking powder, 1 tsp.
- Eggs, 2
- Truvia, .75 c
- Butter, .5 c
- Unsweetened chocolate chips, 1.5 c
- Peanut butter, 1 c
- Unsweetened coconut milk, 2 tbsp.
- Coconut flour, 3 c

What to Do

1. Start by setting your oven to 350.

2. Mix together the salt, coconut, vanilla, cinnamon, egg, butter, chocolate chips, peanut butter, milk, and flour. Make sure that everything is mixed together.

3. Roll the dough into 16 1.5-inch balls.

4. Place the dough on the cookie sheet and slide into the oven. Allow the cookies to bake for 15 minutes. You can adjust the cooking time depending on how soft or crispy you want your cookies.

5. Take the cookies out of the oven and allow them to cool.

6. Keep the cookies in a lidded bowl or a Ziploc bag at room temperature. They will last a week.

Berry Cheesecake

This recipe makes 6 servings and contains 431 calories; 40 g fat; 13 g protein; 3 g net carbs per serving

What You Need

Crust:

- Vanilla, 1 tsp.
- Stevia, 3 tbsp.
- Melted coconut oil, .33 c
- Coconut flour, 2 c

Filling:

- Salt, .5 tsp.
- Vanilla, 1 tsp.
- Lemon juice, 1 tbsp.
- Powdered erythritol, 1.25 c
- Cream cheese, 4 8-oz. pack
- Eggs, 3
- Topping:
- Powdered erythritol
- Mixed berries, 1-2 c

What to Do

1. Start by placing your oven to 350.
2. Mix together the vanilla, stevia, butter, and coconut flours. Grease a springform pan and press the crust into the pan.
3. Bake the crust for ten minutes. Allow the crust to cool for at least ten minutes before putting anything in it.
4. Beat the cream cheese with an electric mixture. Add in the eggs, beating until completely combined.
5. Beat in the salt, vanilla, lemon juice, and powdered erythritol. Mix until completely combined.
6. Pour the filling into the pan and smooth the top out.
7. Place the cheesecake in the oven and bake it for 50 minutes.

8. Carefully remove the cheesecake and cool for 30 minutes. Remove the cake from the pan.

9. Mix the erythritol and berries together and pour over top of the cheesecake.

10. Keep the cake refrigerated, it will last a week.

Chocolate Cake

This recipe makes 6 servings and contains 347 calories; 32 g fat; 9 g protein; 2 g net carbs per serving

What You Need

- Erythritol, 1 c
- Baking powder, 1 tsp.
- Baking soda, 1 tsp.
- Unsweetened coconut milk, .5 c
- Eggs, 6
- Softened butter, .75 c
- Unsweetened cocoa powder, .5 c
- Coconut flour, 3.5 c
- Frosting:
- Salt
- Vanilla, 1 tsp.
- Powdered erythritol, .66 c
- Softened butter, .33 c
- Melted unsweetened chocolate chips, .5 c
- Softened cream cheese, 2 8-oz. packs

What to Do

1. Start by placing your oven to 350.

2. Place parchment in a springform pan.

3. Mix together the erythritol, baking powder, baking soda, coconut milk, eggs, butter, cocoa powder, and coconut flour. Mix until it comes together.

4. Pour this into the springform pan and bake it for 25 minutes. A toothpick should come out clean.

5. Meanwhile, beat together the salt, vanilla, powdered erythritol, butter, and melted chocolate chips.

6. Take the cake out of the oven. Allow it to cool off for a few minutes and then remove it from the pan. Once the cake is completely cooled, spread the frosting over it.

7. The cake will last a week in the refrigerator.

Lemon Bundt Cake

This recipe makes 8 servings and contains 391 calories; 23 g fat; 8 g protein; 5 g net carbs per serving

What You Need

- Salt, .5 tsp.
- Nutmeg, .25 tsp.
- Cinnamon, .5 tsp.
- Vanilla, .5 tsp.
- Baking powder, 1 tsp.
- Baking soda, 1 tsp.
- Raspberries, 2.5 c
- Powdered erythritol, 1 c
- Beaten eggs, 3
- Melted coconut oil, .5 c
- Lemon zest, 3 tsp.
- Coconut milk, 1 c
- Coconut flour, 3 c

What to Do

1. Start by placing your oven to 350.
2. Mix together the salt, nutmeg, cinnamon, vanilla, baking powder, baking soda, erythritol, eggs, coconut oil, lemon zest, coconut milk, and coconut flour. Stir until everything is well combined.
3. Carefully fold the raspberries in.
4. Spray a Bundt pan with cooking spray.
5. Pour the prepared batter into the Bundt pan.
6. Wrap the top of the pan with foil.
7. Slide the pan into the oven and bake it for 20 minutes. A toothpick should come out clean.
8. Allow the Bundt pan to cool off completely and then carefully flip over onto a plate to remove.
9. This will keep for a week at room temperature.

Blueberry Pudding

This recipe makes 6 servings and contains 132 calories; 14 g fat; 4 g protein; 4 g net carbs per serving

What You Need

- Salt
- Vanilla, .25 tsp.
- Lemon juice, 1 tbsp.
- Coconut oil, 2 tbsp.
- Desiccated coconut, 1 c
- Chia seeds, .5 c
- Blueberries, 2 c
- Unsweetened coconut cream, .5 c
- Unsweetened coconut milk, 3 c

What to Do

1. Mix the coconut milk and coconut cream together.

2. Mix in the salt, vanilla, lemon juice, coconut, coconut oil, chia seeds, and blueberries until everything is well combined.

3. Divide the pudding between six containers and refrigerate for at least four hours before servings.

4. This will keep for five days in the refrigerator.

Berry Popsicles

This recipe makes 6 servings and contains 88 calories; 2 g fat; 4 g protein; 2 g net carbs per serving

What You Need

- Liquid stevia, 20-25 drops
- Heavy cream, .25 c
- Sour cream, .25 c
- Unsweetened coconut milk, 1 c
- Coconut oil, .25 c
- Blueberries, 1 c
- Strawberries, 1 c

What to Do

1. Add all of the ingredients to a blender and mix until smooth. You can adjust the sweetness as needed.

2. Pour the mixture through a mesh sieve into a measuring c. Push the mixture through to help clean out the seeds.

3. Pour this into popsicle molds and allow them to freeze at least two hours or until solid.

Chocolate Pudding

This recipe makes 6 servings and contains 198 calories; 17 g fat; 4 g protein; 2 g net carbs per serving

What You Need

- Stevia
- Salt
- Vanilla, .5 tsp.
- Cayenne, .5 tsp.
- Unsweetened coconut milk, 4 tbsp.
- Cinnamon, 4 tsp.
- Unsweetened cacao powder, .5 c
- Avocados, 4

What to Do

1. Place the avocados into a food processor and pulse until they are almost smooth.
2. Add in all of the rest of the ingredients and pulse until they are all mixed and smooth.
3. Pour the mixture into six mason jars. Refrigerate until they are chilled and serve.
4. They will keep in the fridge for three days.

Conclusion

Thanks for making it through to the end of *Keto Meal Prep 2020*. Let's hope it was informative and able to provide you with all of the tools you need to achieve your goals whatever they may be.

I hope that you have found all the information that you need to achieve your keto meal prep goals. You now understand the basics of a ketogenic diet and what it takes to be successful. You can use any of the meal prep plans I provided, or you can use the recipes to create a meal prep plan all on your own.

The important thing to remember is that following a ketogenic diet isn't some fad diet that will fade away with time. It is a lifestyle change that is going to improve your body. The main purpose of this diet is to change your body's fuel source from fat to ketones by reducing your carb intake. After your body has reached ketosis, losing weight won't be as much of a pain.

You now know what it takes to live a healthy and satisfying life. Act now, and use the information found within these pages to make your life healthier and easier. There is no shortage of recipes, either. You will be amazed at how quickly your life and body can change when you start a ketogenic diet.

Finally, if you found this book useful in any way, a review on Amazon is always appreciated!

Description

Have you been struggling to lose those last few pounds? Are you tired of the diets that never seem to help? Do you have a busy life and don't have a lot of time to cook?

If you answered yes to any of these questions, then this book is for you. A ketogenic diet will help you to lose that stubborn weight, and when it's coupled with meal prep, it makes your life easier.

In this book, you will not only learn about keto, but you will also learn about meal prepping and how it can improve your life. You will find:

- Three meal prep plans for beginners, maintenance, and performance
- What the keto diet is
- How to reach ketosis
- How to start meal prepping
- The tools you will need
- Plus lots of recipes
- And much more

Losing weight doesn't have to be hard. You don't have to have a lot of time either. Through meal prepping and keto, you can get healthy and still have time for the rest of your life. Don't wait any longer to change your life for the better. Get this book today and make better choices tomorrow.

30-Day Ketogenic Meal Plan:

The Ultimate Keto Meal Plan to Lose Weight and Be Healthy in 30 Days

Tyler MacDonald

© Copyright 2019 by Tyler MacDonald - All rights reserved.

This book is provided with the sole purpose of providing relevant information on a specific topic for which every reasonable effort has been made to ensure that it is both accurate and reasonable. Nevertheless, by purchasing this book you consent to the fact that the author, as well as the publisher, are in no way experts on the topics contained herein, regardless of any claims as such that may be made within. As such, any suggestions or recommendations that are made within are done so purely for entertainment value. It is recommended that you always consult a professional prior to undertaking any of the advice or techniques discussed within.

This is a legally binding declaration that is considered both valid and fair by both the Committee of Publishers Association and the American Bar Association and should be considered as legally binding within the United States.

The reproduction, transmission, and duplication of any of the content found herein, including any specific or extended information will be done as an illegal act regardless of the end form the information ultimately takes. This includes copied versions of the work physical, digital, and audio unless an expressed consent of the Publisher is provided beforehand. Any additional rights reserved.

Furthermore, the information that can be found within the pages described forthwith shall be considered both accurate and truthful when it comes to the recounting of facts. As such, any use, correct or incorrect, of the provided information will render the Publisher free of responsibility as to the actions taken outside of their direct purview. Regardless, there are zero scenarios where the original author or the Publisher can be deemed liable in any fashion for any damages or hardships that may result from any of the information discussed herein.

Additionally, the information in the following pages is intended only for informational purposes and should thus be thought of as universal. As befitting its nature, it is presented without assurance regarding its prolonged validity or interim quality. Trademarks that are mentioned are done without written consent and can in no way be considered an endorsement from the trademark holder.

Introduction

First off, thank you for choosing *30-Day Ketogenic Meal Plan*. This is your first step along the path of weight loss and a healthy lifestyle. I'm sure this isn't an easy first step either. The worthwhile steps never are, but you took it.

It's tough when you have a busy schedule and life to find time to make smart choices. When you add in a new diet, that makes life even more difficult. The thing is, it doesn't have to be that way. With some careful planning, you can lose weight, get healthy, and still accomplish everything else that you want.

The first thing you have to do is figure out the things you can and cannot eat when following a ketogenic diet. Then, you find a bunch of recipes, calculate your macros, and create a meal plan. That's it. Once you have come up with that meal plan, you write down a grocery list of things that you need and go get it.

But, I understand it's easier said than done. It can be frustrating to do all of that on your own, especially if you will be following a new diet. That's what this book is here to help you. You will find all of the recipes you need and tips on how to create your own meal plan. The best part, though, is there is a 30-day plan within these pages.

In those 30 days, you will lose weight, reach ketosis, and see amazing results. You will also get a good understanding of what it's like to be in a ketogenic diet. That means when those 30 days are up, you will feel confident enough to create your own meal plans so that you stick with the diet and continue to get healthy.

The meal plan is going to jumpstart your journey. Plus, you will find more recipes that you can use for the meal plans you will create. That means this book contains more than just the recipes used in the 30-day meal plan.

I am very excited for you to continue on your weight loss journey. You will discover a lot about yourself along the way, and I'm certain you will enjoy every minute of it. I want you to commit to yourself right now that you will follow this 30-day meal plan. Trust me; you won't regret it.

The Basics

The ketogenic diet isn't just a popular diet of today. It is easy to stick with and help you feel better overall. With this diet, you eat low carbs, moderate protein, and high fats. By doing this, your body learns to burn your fat stores instead of carbs for fuel. Burning fat creates more energy to get you through your day. You will soon have more energy than you have ever had in your life. This diet helps you lose weight and get rid of fat.

Your body's fat stores get converted into fatty acids that are used in the liver. They then get pushed through the body as ketones that are used as glucose sugar rather than artificial sugar.

This allows the body to grow and repair itself better. It also gives the body more calories to burn for energy without having to eat as much.

The most important thing you need to know about this diet is the way ketosis works. Ketosis is the main structure of this diet.

Once the body gets into the state of ketosis, it means the body will break down the fat stores to give your body the energy it needs. This means the body is giving itself a way to use the fats you eat rather than depending on the carbs you eat. You might still be wondering what the ketogenic diet is, let's dig a bit deeper and find out.

This diet was developed in the 1920s to treat epilepsy. This diet stopped being used when pharmaceutical companies developed anti-seizure medication. Now, 70 years later, doctors have rediscovered it as a better alternative than medicine. It has become more popular and is constantly receiving attention in the media for the numerous problems it can treat.

The Principles

When you learn more about foods that are keto-friendly and are used to living a keto life, it will be easy for you to know how much and what you need to eat. Here is what your daily macros, fats, proteins, and carbs need to look like.

- *Carbohydrates*

Everybody's carbs tolerance will be different. The challenge is finding your "ideal" intake. When starting this diet, begin with a very low level of carb to make sure you get into ketosis fast. This is the state where your body makes the ketones. A goal would be around 20 grams of carbs each day. The best way to measure blood ketones is with a blood ketone meter. These let you measure your ketones after three days of following the keto lifestyle. You can also use urine strips to measure your ketones, but these aren't as accurate. Begin adding carbs around five grams per week until you can barely detect extremely low levels of ketones. This is the most reliable way to figure out your limit of carbs. You can easily find urine strips or blood ketone meters online.

- *Protein*

How much protein you should consume can be figured out by activity level and body weight. People that are more active will need more protein during the day as compared to those who have a sedentary lifestyle. A better estimate for people who have high body fat could be figured by subtracting the amount of protein you eat from the lean body mass. This is figured by subtracting body fat from body weight.

Eating enough protein is great to build or preserve muscle mass. If you eat too much protein, you could knock yourself out of ketosis since your body converts excess protein into glycogen.

- *How Much Protein?*

If you know your weight in pounds, just multiply that by 0.6 to get the lowest number of grams of protein you need to consume every day. To find the largest amount, you have to figure out your weight in grams and multiply that by your weight in pounds. If you know your weight in kilograms, multiply that by 1.3 or 2.2. This rule will apply to most people, but athletes will have higher protein requirements. You need to eat the least amount of protein to keep from losing muscle mass while dieting. If you are very active, you need to eat as close to your top limit as possible.

- *Fat: 60 to 75 percent*

Your fat intake makes up the rest of your energy needs. It is the filler to your energy requirements. Fat intake will be different for everyone, and it depends on what your goals are. You don't even need to count your calories or fat intake while following a keto diet because normally you won't overeat. When you eat foods that are low carb, a moderate amount of protein, and high in fats will keep you feeling fuller longer. Studies show that fats and protein are the most filling nutrients while carbs aren't. Fat gives you a lot of energy without spiking your insulin. This is why you shouldn't have any cravings while following this diet. You shouldn't suffer and mood or energy swings like you would on a low fat, calorie restricted diet.

Guidelines

Here are some great ways to help you stay in ketosis and get the most from your ketogenic diet. These tips will help you through the "keto flu." In the first few days or weeks while your body transitions into ketosis, you might feel dizzy, sluggish, or tired.

- *Macros*

You need to be sure you stick with your macros. The normal 10 percent carbs, 20 percent protein, and 70 percent fats should be followed simply because it works. If you eat too many carbs, you aren't going to be burning fat. If you eat too much protein, it isn't going to get burned because you aren't using it. If you don't eat enough fats, you aren't going to feel full. All of this will add up to less energy. These ratios let you eat whole foods to get into ketosis, and this includes lots of leafy green vegetables that help to break down meats.

- *Electrolytes*

Make sure you keep plenty of electrolytes in your system. Electrolytes are minerals in the blood that keeps the body hydrated and help the muscles and nerves work in unison. When your body begins producing ketones, it will flush out more water, and this depletes the body's supply of electrolytes. What this means for you is you need to increase the amount of salt in your diet since your body can't retain sodium. Many keto followers fix this problem by drinking bouillon or bone broth each day. This is especially true during the first few weeks on this diet while the body gets adjusted. If you begin to feel achy while your body goes through carb withdrawals, bouillon will help. Other keto followers will take magnesium supplements, too.

- *Water*

You need to drink more water than normal. Everybody says you need to drink water, but no one takes it seriously until they get kidney stones. Drinking no less than 64 ounces of water every day is going to make your body feel hydrated, full, and clean. It also helps keep your bowels working correctly. If you are looking to lose weight while on this diet, water will help you with this, too.

- *Track Your Eating*

You need to measure what you eat. By doing this, it can turn this diet into a game. You can find apps that will help you measure your macros and track your meals daily. A specific app called Quip helps you make shopping lists. It has check marks that let you use your shopping list over and over again.

- *Calories*

You need to make sure you eat all your calories. You can't do a low-calorie diet along with a ketogenic diet. If you do this, your body won't be able to fuel itself. Fat is now what fuels your body. Without eating the correct amounts, you are going to feel hungry, and you aren't going to lose any weight. Most people who follow the keto diet eat between 1,800 and 2,000 calories each day. You might realize that eating less isn't going to help you lose weight; it might actually stall any weight loss. You can't binge eat, either. You aren't going to lose weight if you eat 5,000 calories each day.

- *Healthy Fats*

You need to have a lot of healthy fats on hand. Fat is considered a bad word in society today. What most people don't realize is there are a lot of good fats out there. Cook your foods in coconut oil or olive oil. Stay away from oils such as corn, soybean, sunflower seed, and vegetable oils. These are all high in omega 6s that cause inflammation. They can actually destroy the omega 3s that are in your body.

- *Whole Foods*

You need to buy whole foods and stay away from anything that says "low carb" on the label. If you look at the label on anything labeled as "low carb", you are going to be shocked at what is in them. Most of it is additives that can't be pronounced. You get to control what goes into your body when you make your meals at home and stick to eating whole foods.

Creating a Meal Plan

If you would like to know how to make your own meal plan, here is a guide you can follow:

- *Make a draft*

Think about what foods you enjoy eating and see if they are on the approved list. Go from there and create your own diet plan. Remember to include lots of healthy fats, a moderate amount of protein, and low carbs.

- *Check*

Go through the recipes you've put into your meal plan to see if the carbs, proteins, and fats match your body weight. If they don't, readjust the meal plan.

- *Research*

Before you begin making a meal plan, research various keto meal plans and see how they measure up. Make sure you go through this whole guide since you don't want to jump in blind.

- *Revise*

Make any changes you need to make and revise any recipes that need to be made better.

- *Discuss*

If you are not sure about anything, talk with an expert. If you still aren't sure, follow the meal plan below or ask other people who have done this diet.

- *Repair*

Look for any improvements that are needed and make any changes that you need to. Be sure it matches your percentage needs of 10/20/70.

- *Follow through*

If you are ready, let's get started.

Here are some tips that will help you be successful when following your meal plan:

- Realize that diets aren't good for everyone. Be sure your diet plan and recipes match your requirements. Make any adjustments and make the portions smaller if needed. If you go over your protein intake, don't worry too much. Just adjust and keep moving forward. If you realize your diet doesn't include enough fats, this can be easily remedied by adding oil or butter to meals.

- Substitute lamb, pork, and fish for each other in recipes because their nutritional values are similar.

- Don't eat unless you are hungry. If you don't feel hungry at mealtime, don't eat. It is perfectly fine to skip a meal.

- Try skipping snacks. You should feel full from your three main meals. If you don't, keep some keto-friendly snack at hand.

- Swap meals: You can swap up your meals during the day. You can eat breakfast for dinner or lunch for breakfast or dinner for lunch. What you eat depends on you.

- Cook your meal. When you cook your own meals, you can control what goes into them. Freeze any uneaten portions or save half and eat it later.

While you are adapting to the ketogenic lifestyle and making your own meal plans, watch out for the following. These are usually sold with fillers and added sugars. Check labels before you buy products and don't forget to calculate your net carbs by subtracting fiber from the total carbs. You want to purchase items that have low net carbs.

- Sliced cheese, especially American can have around three carbs for each slice. Stick with shredded cheese that contains no fillers. You will be eating less than one carb per serving.

- Salad dressing: these might have a lot of sugar in them, look for ones that have around one net carb for each serving.

- Sugar-free: Just because something is labeled as "sugar-free" doesn't mean it will be low carb. Anything that is labeled as "gluten-free" will never equal low carb. Low carb doesn't mean it will be ketogenic. You could find 20 to 30 carbs in a bagel that is labeled as low carb.

- Frozen burgers: Most frozen foods use fillers and could carry between three and five carbs per burger. If you made them yourself, it could be zero carbs.

- Deli foods: Grocery stores make it easy to walk in and be able to grab a quick bite to eat. Even though these are made each day, they usually include breading and sugars you won't be able to see just by looking at them.

- Whey protein: This powder might be very high in sugar. Check the label to find some no or low-carb varieties.

- Coconut milk: This contains good fats but does contain about one net carb for unsweetened. The sweetened variety has about nine carbs per serving.

- Tomato sauce: When looking for tomato sauce in the grocery store, you will see there will be anywhere between 10 and 20 net carbs in each serving. Try to find ones that don't have any added sugars and are less than four net carbs for each serving.

- Dairy products: Again, look at the labels. Most cream cheese, sour cream, and heavy whipping cream will have around two to three net carbs for each serving. Organic brands won't have any carbs or under one net carb.

- Peanut butter: Most brands of peanut butter will contain a lot of sugar. Find a brand that has low net carbs. The organic brands will contain very low or no sugar.

Sticking with the Diet

There are various ways to help you stick with a diet. Most people will give up after some time, and it is mainly because normal diets make them give up foods that they like eating. The keto diet requires you to give up many foods you like, but this is mainly just carbs. This makes it easier to stay on and maintain. Here are some tips to make sure you stay healthy while following this diet for a long time.

- Don't let yourself get hungry. Many times, if you let yourself get too hungry, you will eat carb-heavy foods that fill you up fast. It can make you have poor judgment when it comes to deciding what you want to eat. You might pick something that won't be good for your new lifestyle.

- Eat vegetables or berries for a snack. If you get hungry between meals, have a handful of nuts, berries, or veggies for a snack. These are nutritious and healthy options that take the place of cupcakes or cookies.

- Make sure you get enough sleep. Studies show that you eat more when you are tired. This produces a hormone that will trick you into thinking you are hungry.

- Drink water. Water doesn't just flush toxins out of your body, but it keeps you hydrated, too. It could also distract you from whatever craving you might be having.

- Find recipes you want to try that are in your diet's guidelines. When you have various foods to taste and sample, it will be easier to stick with your diet since you are eating a variety of foods and it won't become boring.

- Try new things and create new recipes. Use foods you know you can eat and try to make new recipes. Being able to play around and experiment will keep your food interesting.

- Create an achievable goal. Having clear goals will motivate you to make sure you reach it.

- Take vitamins and supplements if you need them. Talk with your doctor first if you think you have a deficiency. Then if they say it is fine, take a supplement

- Find an accountability partner. If you have somebody you have to report to and will support your progress, it will help you stay on track. Find somebody who will support you mentally as well as physically.

30-Day Meal Plan

The 30-Day Meal Plan is broken down into four weeks. Every day has a snack option. Now, you can choose to eat the snack between lunch and dinner, or you can have the snack as a dessert after dinner. If there is a day where you don't feel like you want a snack or dessert, that's perfectly fine. You don't have to eat one.

Week One	Breakfast	Lunch	Snack	Dinner
Day 1	Avocado Milkshake	Chicken Wraps	Cinnamon Smoothie	Cauliflower Mac & Cheese
Day 2	Granola	Cauliflower Soup	Blueberry Smoothie	Turkey Meatloaf
Day 3	Peanut Butter Smoothie	Grilled Salmon with Asparagus	Dark Chocolate	Lettuce Wrap Cheeseburger
Day 4	Cream Cheese Pancakes	Cauliflower Soup (leftovers)	Vanilla Ice Cream	Grilled Salmon with Asparagus (leftovers)
Day 5	Keto Coffee	Turkey Meatloaf (leftovers)	Bacon Deviled Eggs	Haddock
Day 6	Lemon Smoothie	Haddock (leftovers)	Dark Chocolate	Pork Loin with Mustard Sauce
Day 7	Bacon and Eggs	Taco Salad	Parmesan Chips	Pork Loin with Mustard Sauce (leftovers)

Week Two	Breakfast	Lunch	Snack	Dinner
Day 8	Breakfast Bake	Crab Salad Avocado	Kale Chips	Zucchini Gratin
Day 9	Peanut Butter Smoothie	Tuna Salad	Parmesan Chips	Thai Chicken Soup
Day 10	Keto Coffee	Zucchini Gratin (leftovers)	Mixed Berries	Bacon Cheese Burger Soup
Day 11	Breakfast Bake (leftovers)	Thai Chicken Soup (leftovers)	Dark Chocolate	Tuna Salad (leftovers)
Day 12	Green Smoothie	Chicken Bacon Burger	Parmesan Chips	Lamb with Sun-Dried Tomatoes
Day 13	Keto Coffee	BLT Salad	Brownies	Thai Lettuce Wrap
Day 14	Avocado and Eggs	Lamb with Sun-Dried Tomatoes (leftovers)	Brownies	Bacon Cheese Burger Soup (leftovers)

Week Three	Breakfast	Lunch	Snack	Dinner
Day 15	Berry Shake	Salmon Salad	Nut Butter and Veggies	Cheesy Broccoli Soup
Day 16	Breakfast Crème	Feta Salad	Cinnamon Smoothie	Cauliflower Soup
Day 17	Lemon Smoothie	Cheesy Broccoli Soup (leftovers)	Brownies	Salmon Salad (leftovers)
Day 18	Avocado and Eggs	Bolognese Zoodles	Dark Chocolate	Cauliflower Soup (leftovers)

Day 19	Cream Cheese Pancakes	Grilled Salmon with Asparagus	Pork Rinds	Cheeseburger
Day 20	Keto Coffee	Cheesy Broccoli Soup (leftovers)	Bacon Fat Bombs	Chicken Bacon Burger
Day 21	Keto Coffee	Feta Salad (leftovers)	Parmesan Chips	Grilled Salmon with Asparagus (leftovers)

Week Four	Breakfast	Lunch	Snack	Dinner
Day 22	Green Smoothie	Zesty Tilapia	Blueberry Muffin	Tri-Tip
Day 23	Peanut Butter Smoothie	Avocado Pesto Zoodles	Pecan Peanut Butter Bars	Sausage Casserole
Day 24	Keto Coffee	Roasted Chicken Thighs with Veggies	Beef Jerky	Zesty Tilapia (leftovers)
Day 25	Chia Berry Smoothie Bowl	Avocado Pesto Zoodles (leftovers)	Peanut Butter Smoothie	Sausage Crust Pizza
Day 26	Blueberry Muffin (leftover)	Sausage Casserole (leftovers)	Peanut Butter Cookies	Garlic Parmesan Salmon
Day 27	Keto Coffee	Zesty Tilapia (leftovers)	Dark Chocolate	Coconut Lime Skirt Steak
Day 28	Bacon and Eggs	Turkey Avocado Salad	Blueberry Muffin	Roasted Chicken Thighs with Veggies (leftovers)
Day 29	Keto Coffee	Garlic Parmesan Salmon (leftovers)	Peanut Butter Smoothie	Coconut Lime Skirt Steak (leftovers)

| Day 30 | Goat Cheese Omelet | Turkey Avocado Salad (leftovers) | Peanut Butter Cookies | Creamy Butter Chicken |

Breakfast

Avocado Milkshake

This recipe makes 1 serving, and contains 437 calories; 43 grams fat; 4 grams protein; 10 grams net carbohydrates per serving

What You Need

- Ice cubes, 5
- Liquid stevia, 5 drops
- Unsweetened coconut milk, .5 c
- Avocado, .5

What to Do

- Simply place the ingredients in your blender and mix until it reaches a smooth consistency.

Granola

This recipe makes 8 servings, and contains 391 calories; 38 grams fat; 10 grams protein; 4 grams net carbohydrates per serving

What You Need

- Sunflower seeds, 1 c
- Sliced almonds, 1 c
- Nutmeg, .5 tsp.
- Cinnamon, 1 tsp.
- Liquid stevia, 10 drops
- Shredded unsweetened coconut, 2 c

- Melted coconut oil, .5 c
- Walnuts, .5 c
- Pumpkin seeds, .5 c

What to Do

- Start by placing your oven on 250. Place parchment paper on two baking sheets and place to the side.
- Toss the walnuts, pumpkin seeds, sunflower seeds, almonds, and shredded coconut together.
- Blend together the nutmeg, cinnamon, stevia, and coconut oil.
- Pour the coconut oil over the nut mixture and toss everything together using your hands. Make sure everything is well coated.
- Spread the granola out between the two baking sheets.
- Slide this in the oven and let it bake for an hour. Every 10-15 minutes, the mixture needs to be stirred to make sure that it browns evenly on all sides.
- Pour the granola in a bowl and allow it to cool off before storing.

Peanut Butter Smoothie

This recipe makes 2 servings, and contains 486 calories; 40 grams fat; 30 grams protein; 6 grams net carbohydrates per serving

What You Need

- Ice cubes, 3
- Peanut butter, 2 tbsp.
- Chocolate protein powder, 1 scoop
- Coconut cream, .75 c
- Water, 1 c

What to Do

- Simply place the ingredients to a blender and mix until it reaches a smooth consistency. Divide into two glasses and serve.

Cream Cheese Pancakes

This recipe makes 1 serving, and contains 365 calories; 29 grams fat; 17 grams protein; 5 grams net carbohydrates per serving

What You Need

- Packet stevia
- Cinnamon, .5 tsp.
- Coconut flour, 1 tbsp.
- Cream cheese, 2 oz.
- Eggs, 2

What to Do

- Place everything in a bowl and beat everything together until it forms a smooth batter.
- Add some butter to a skillet and once melted, spoon in some of the batter. Cook until bubbles start to form on the pancake, flip, and cook for a few minutes more.
- Continue until the batter is used.
- Serve with some sugar-free syrup and butter.

Keto Coffee

This recipe makes 1 serving, and contains 284 calories; 24 grams fat; 16 grams protein; 0 gram net carbohydrates per serving

What You Need

- Vanilla, .25 tsp.
- Coconut oil, 1 tbsp.
- Butter, 1 tbsp.

- Brewed coffee, 1 c

What to Do

- Add your hot coffee to a blender along with all of the other ingredients. Blend until mixed and frothy. Enjoy.

Lemon Smoothie

This recipe makes 1 serving, and contains 503 calories; 45 grams fat; 29 grams protein; 11 grams net carbohydrates per serving

What You Need

- Sweetener, 1 tsp.
- Coconut oil, 1 tbsp.
- Plain protein powder, 1 tsp.
- Lemon juice, .25 c
- Heavy cream, .25 c
- Unsweetened cashew milk, 1 c

What to Do

- Simply place the ingredients to a blender and mix until it forms a smooth consistency. Divide into a glass and enjoy.

Breakfast Bake

This recipe makes 8 servings, and contains 303 calories; 24 grams fat; 17 grams protein; 3 grams net carbohydrates per serving

What You Need

- Sausage, 1 lb.
- Eggs, 8

- Olive oil, 1 tbsp.
- Shredded cheddar, .5 c
- Pepper
- Salt
- Chopped fresh oregano, 1 tbsp.
- Cooked spaghetti squash, 2 c

What to Do

- Start by placing your oven to 375. Grease a baking dish with some oil and place to the side.
- Heat up the olive oil in a large skillet.
- Add in the sausage and brown. This will take about five minutes. Break apart as you cook. Beat the eggs, oregano, and squash together in a bowl. Season with a bit of pepper and salt.
- Mix the sausage into the eggs and pour into the baking dish.
- Sprinkle the cheese over the casserole and then wrap the dish with foil.
- Slide this in the oven for 30 minutes. Take it out of the oven and remove the foil. Slide back in and cook for another 15 minutes.
- Allow the casserole to cool for ten minutes before serving.

Green Smoothie

This recipe makes 2 servings, and contains 436 calories; 36 grams fat; 28 grams protein; 6 grams net carbohydrates per serving

What You Need

- Vanilla protein powder, 1 scoop
- Coconut oil, 1 tbsp.
- Cream cheese, .75 c
- Shredded kale, .5 c
- Blueberries, .5 c

- Water, 1 c

What to Do

- Simply place the ingredients to a blender and process until it reaches a smooth consistency.
- Divide into two glasses and enjoy.

Avocado and Eggs

This recipe makes 4 servings, and contains 324 calories; 25 grams fat; 19 grams protein; 3 grams net carbohydrates per serving

What You Need

- Halved and pitted avocado, 2
- Pepper
- Salt
- Cheddar cheese, .25 c
- Shredded cooked chicken breast, 4 oz
- Eggs, 4

What to Do

- Start by placing your oven to 425.
- Hollow out the avocado halves until the holes left by the pit is about twice the size it was.
- Lay the avocado halves in a baking dish with the cut side up.
- Break an egg into each half and then top each with some of the chicken, cheese, and some pepper and salt.
- Bake these for 15-20 minutes. Serve.

Berry Shake

This recipe makes 2 servings, and contains 330 calories; 29 grams fat; 2 grams protein; 12 grams net carbohydrates per serving

What You Need

- Frozen strawberries, .5 c
- Frozen raspberries, .5 c
- Frozen blueberries, .5 c
- Vanilla, 1 tsp.
- Unsweetened coconut milk, 1 c
- Ice cubes

What to Do

- Simply add everything to your blender and mix until it forms a smooth consistency.
- Pour the shake into two glasses and serve.

Breakfast Crème

This recipe makes 1 serving, and contains 470 calories; 36 grams fat; 28 grams protein; 7 grams net carbohydrates per serving

What You Need

- Vanilla, .25 tsp.
- Cinnamon, .25
- Butter, 1 tsp.
- Ricotta, 1 c

What to Do

- Place everything in a microwave safe bowl. Mix together and then microwave for a minute. Stir again and serve.

Chia Berry Smoothie Bowl

This recipe makes 3 servings, and contains 401 calories; 39 grams fat; 3 grams protein; 9 grams net carbohydrates per serving

What You Need

- Liquid stevia, 3 drops
- Vanilla, 1 tsp.
- Chia seeds, 2 tbsp.
- MCT oil, 2 tbsp.
- Frozen mixed berries, 1 c
- Full-fat coconut milk, 1.5 c
- Optional Toppings:
- Almonds
- Shredded coconut
- Fresh berries

What to Do

- Add all of the ingredients, except for the chia seeds, to your blender and mix until it forms a smooth consistency. Pour into a lidded container and stir in the chia seeds.
- Allow this to refrigerate overnight. It will thicken up.
- When you are ready to eat, top with your favorite toppings.

Goat Cheese Omelet

This recipe makes 4 servings, and contains 506 calories; 43 grams fat; 24 grams protein; 4 grams net carbohydrates per serving

What You Need

- Pepper
- Salt
- Chopped scallions, .25 c
- Heavy cream, 4 tbsp.
- Goat cheese, 8 oz.
- Butter, 2 tbsp.
- Spinach, 6 c
- Dijon, 1 tsp.
- Olive oil, 2 tsp.
- Eggs, 8

What to Do

- Add two teaspoons of oil to a skillet and add in the spinach. Cook until the spinach has wilted, about one to two minutes. Stir in the salt, pepper, and mustard.
- Take the spinach out of the pan and place to the side.
- Beat together the pepper, salt, cream, and eggs.
- Add the butter to the skillet and melt.
- Pour a quarter of the egg mixture into the skillet and allow the egg to set a bit. Spread a quarter of the spinach and goat cheese over the egg.
- Cook for a few more minutes, flip, and then fold the omelet in half once the egg is completely set.
- Continue with the rest of the eggs, making a total of four omelets.
- Garnish the omelets with scallions.

Blueberry Muffin

This recipe makes 15 servings, and contains 147 calories; 13 grams fat; 5 grams protein; 3 grams net carbohydrates per serving

What You Need

- Melted butter, 2 tbsp.
- Fresh blueberries, 4 oz.
- Eggs, 2
- Salt, .5 tsp.
- Sour cream, 1 c
- Erythritol, .25 c
- Baking soda, .5 tsp.
- Almond flour, 2 c

What to Do

- Start by placing your oven to 350. Like a cupcake tin with paper liners, or use silicone molds.
- Whisk together the almond flour, baking soda, and erythritol together.
- Beat the eggs lightly and mix in the sour cream and butter. Make sure it is completely combined.
- Pour the sour cream mixture into the almond flour mixture. Stir until completely mixed. Fold in the blueberries.
- Divide the batter between the prepared cupcake tin holes, filling them halfway full.
- Bake the muffins for 20 minutes. They should be golden.
- Allow the cupcakes to cool slightly. Serve warm with a bit of butter.

Cinnamon Chia Pudding

This recipe makes 1 serving, and contains 384 calories; 24 grams fat; 16 grams protein; 28 grams net carbohydrates per serving

What You Need

- Liquid stevia, 8 drops
- Peanut butter, 1 tbsp.

- Cinnamon, .5 tsp.
- Unsweetened almond milk, 1 c
- Chia seeds, 1 tbsp.

What to Do

- Add everything except for the chia seeds to your blender and mix until smooth.
- Add this to a bowl and then mix in the chia seeds. Stir everything together and let it refrigerate for at least three hours. Enjoy.

Cacao Chia Shake

This recipe makes 1 serving, and contains 533 calories; 37 grams fat; 15 grams protein; 12 grams net carbohydrates per serving

What You Need

- Ice cubes, 5
- Unsweetened almond milk, 1 c
- 80-100% dark chocolate, .5 oz.
- Chia seeds, 1 tbsp.
- Avocado, .5

What to Do

- Stir the almond milk and chia seeds together and allow this to sit for ten minutes.
- Now, place everything in your blender and mix until smooth.
- Pour into a glass and top with some extra dark chocolate.

Everything Bagel

This recipe makes 12 servings, and contains 25 calories; 2 grams fat; 3 grams protein; 1 gram net carbohydrates per serving

What You Need

- Everything bagel seasoning
- Full-fat cream cheese, 4 oz.
- Smoked salmon, 4 oz.
- Full-fat butter, 1 tbsp.

What to Do

- Add the cream cheese, salmon, and butter to a bowl and mix everything together until everything is well mixed. Make sure that you don't have clumps of ingredients. You want it to be very smooth.
- Allow this to refrigerate for 30 minutes. This will let the mixture stiffen up some so that you can work with it better.
- Once the mixture is a little firmer, divide it out into 12 portions and roll them into balls.
- Pour the bagel seasoning in a bowl and roll the balls in the seasonings. Press the seasoning into the balls so that it sticks.
- If you don't like the taste of salmon, you can use cooked and crumbled bacon instead.
- Once you have the bagels made, keep them refrigerated. This will allow them to stay firmer so that you can grab one and go when you don't have time to cook in the morning.

Egg Muffin Cup

This recipe makes 1 serving, and contains 294 calories; 25 grams fat; 13 grams protein; 3 grams net carbohydrates per serving

What You Need

- Pepper
- Salt
- Egg, 1
- Grated parmesan, 3 tbsp.
- Sun-dried tomatoes, 1 tbsp. – chopped

- Butter, 1 tbsp.
- Diced veggies of choice, .33 c

What to Do

- Place one tablespoon butter into a microwave-safe mug. Put your vegetables of choice into the bottom of the mug. Put in microwave and cook one minute on high power if veggies are precooked. If the veggies are raw, cook for three minutes.
- Add in the spinach, cheese, and one egg. Stir well to combine everything. Sprinkle with pepper and salt, stir again. Microwave one more minute.

Latkes

This recipe makes 8 servings, and contains 252 calories; 21 grams fat; 5 grams protein; 4 grams net carbohydrates per serving

What You Need

- Coconut oil, 4 tbsp.
- Pepper
- Marjoram, 2 tsp.
- Psyllium husk powder, 1 tbsp.
- Flax meal, .25 c
- Egg, 1
- Sliced onion, 1 small
- Salt
- Rutabaga, 1 medium

What to Do

- Wash and peel the rutabaga. Use a spiralizer to make noodles. A julienne peeler will also work if you don't have a spiralizer. Put the rutabaga into a colander with half teaspoon salt and let sit for 20 minutes.
- Let all the moisture drain from the rutabaga. If there is any moisture left, use paper towels to blot remaining moisture.

- Place the onion and rutabaga into a bowl along with marjoram, psyllium powder, flax meal, and egg. Sprinkle with pepper and salt and mix well.

- Place a skillet on medium heat and melt the coconut oil. Place spoonfuls of the mixture into the skillet to make about four latkes at one time. Flatten each with a spatula. Cook ten minutes per side until browned well.

- Add more coconut as needed until all mixture is used up. Once everything is cooked, enjoy.

Mushroom Frittata

This recipe makes 6 servings, and contains 316 calories; 27 grams fat; 16 grams protein; 1 gram net carbohydrates per serving

What You Need

- Pepper
- Salt
- Crumbled goat cheese, .5 c
- Eggs, 10
- Sliced bacon, 6
- Shredded spinach, 1 c
- Sliced mushrooms, 1 c
- Olive oil, 2 tbsp.

What to Do

- You need to warm your oven to 350.
- Cook the bacon in a large skillet. When crisp, take out and drain.
- In the same skillet, add the oil and heat.
- Add mushrooms and sauté until browned.
- When the bacon is cool enough, crumble and add to the skillet along with the spinach until spinach is wilted.
- Crack eggs into a bowl and beat slightly. Pour into skillet. Lift the edges of the eggs, so the uncooked eggs flow underneath for about four minutes.

- Sprinkle top with goat cheese and season with pepper and salt.
- Place into the oven and bake 15 minutes.
- Take out of the oven and allow to stand for five minutes.
- Cut into six wedges and enjoy.

Artichoke and Bacon Omelet

This recipe makes 4 servings, and contains 435 calories; 39 grams fat; 17 grams protein; 3 grams net carbohydrates per serving

What You Need

- Pepper
- Salt
- Chopped artichoke hearts, .5 c
- Chopped onion, .25 c
- Olive oil, 1 tbsp.
- Sliced bacon, 8
- Heavy cream, 2 tbsp.
- Eggs, 6

What to Do

- Place a skillet on medium heat and cook bacon. When bacon is crisp, take out, and drain. Once you can handle the bacon, crumble.
- Add into a bowl along with heavy cream and eggs. Whisk until well blended.
- In the same pan, add the oil and onion. Cook until softened.
- Pour eggs into skillet. Cook, lifting edges of egg to allow uncooked portions to flow under. Do this for about two minutes.
- Sprinkle artichoke hearts on top and gently turn the omelet over. Cook another four minutes, until egg is set. Flip over one more time, so artichokes are on top.
- Take off heat, slice into quarters, season with pepper and salt. Put onto plates and enjoy.

Caprese Omelet

This recipe makes 2 servings, and contains 258 calories; 43 grams fat; 33 grams protein; 4 grams net carbohydrates per serving

What You Need

- Shredded mozzarella, 5 oz.
- Chopped basil, 1 tbsp.
- Halved cherry tomatoes, 3 oz.
- Pepper
- Olive oil, 2 tbsp.
- Salt
- Eggs, 6

What to Do

- Break eggs into a bowl, sprinkle with pepper and salt. Whisk well to combine. Add in the basil. Stir well.
- Place a skillet on top of the stove and heat on medium. Add tomatoes and fry for some time. Take the tomatoes out of the skillet. Pour the eggs into the skillet and add the tomatoes to the top. Let cook until eggs are slightly firm. Add cheese to the top.
- Turn down heat and cook until eggs are totally set. Take out of the pan and serve.

Lunch

Chicken Wraps

This recipe makes 4 servings, and contains 264 calories; 20 grams fat; 12 grams protein; 6 grams net carbohydrates per serving

What You Need

- Chopped avocado, .5
- Chopped walnuts, .25 c
- Large lettuce leaves, 8
- Pepper
- Salt
- Chopped cooked chicken breast, 6 oz.
- Chopped fresh thyme, 2 tsp.
- Lemon juice, 1 tsp.
- Mayonnaise, .33 c

What to Do

- Mix the thyme, lemon juice, mayonnaise, and avocado together.
- Mix the chicken into the mixture along with some pepper and salt.
- Divide the chicken mixture between the lettuce leaves and top with some walnuts.
- Each person gets two wraps.

Grilled Salmon and Asparagus

This recipe makes 4 servings, and contains 607 calories; 26 grams fat; 82 grams protein; 3 grams net carbohydrates per serving

What You Need

- Lemon juice, .5 tsp.
- Salmon, 4 fillets
- Garlic salt, 1 tsp.
- Pepper, .5 tsp.
- Crushed garlic, 4 cloves
- Asparagus, 1 lb.
- Basil, 2 tbsp.
- Softened butter, .25 c

What to Do

- Add the butter to a small pot, melt, and add in the garlic. Cook this for about two minutes and then discard the garlic.
- Add two tablespoons of butter onto the salmon and rub all over the fillets, making sure you coat both sides.
- Lay the salmon onto a preheated grill and cook for four minutes.
- After the first side is cooked, lay the asparagus on the grill and flip the salmon. Cook everything for another four minutes. The salmon is cooked through with it flakes easily with a fork.
- To serve, add on the rest of the butter, pepper, garlic salt, and lemon juice onto the fish.

Chicken Bacon Burger

This recipe makes 6 servings, and contains 374 calories; 33 grams fat; 18 grams protein; 1 gram net carbohydrates per serving

What You Need

- Sliced avocado
- Large lettuce leaves, 6
- Coconut oil, 2 tbsp.
- Pepper

- Salt
- Chopped basil, 1 tsp.
- Ground almonds, .25 c
- Chopped bacon, 8 slices
- Ground chicken, 1 lb.

What to Do

- Start by placing your oven to 350. Line a baking sheet with some parchment.
- Mix together the pepper, salt, basil, almonds, bacon, and chicken.
- Form the meat mixture into six patties.
- Add the coconut oil to a skillet. Add the patties to the pan and sear on both sides, about three minutes on both sides.
- Lay the patties on the baking sheet and cook them for 15 minutes, or until they are cooked through.
- Serve the burgers on a lettuce leaf and topped with some avocado.

Bolognese Zoodles

This recipe makes 4 servings, and contains 565 calories; 38 grams fat; 46 grams protein; 5 grams net carbohydrates per serving

What You Need

- Parmesan, .25 c
- Water, .25 c
- Crushed tomatoes, 1 can
- Oregano, 1 tsp.
- Pepper, .25 tsp.
- Salt, 1 tsp.
- Tomato paste, 2 tbsp.
- Butter, 3 tbsp.

- Basil, 1 tsp.
- Ground beef, 1.5 lbs.
- Minced garlic, 3 cloves
- Chopped celery, 1 stalk
- Chopped small onion
- Spiralized zucchini, 4

What to Do

- Spiralize the zucchinis and lay them out on a paper towel.
- Melt the butter in a pan and cook the onion and celery. Cook until the onions become translucent, around three minutes.
- Mix in the garlic and sauté everything together until fragrant.
- Mix the ground beef and cook until browned.
- Mix in the water, pepper, salt, oregano, basil, crushed tomatoes, and tomato paste. Allow this to come up to a boil.
- Turn the heat down and cook for about ten to 12 minutes. Everything should thicken up and be well combined.
- Mix in the zoodles and allow the mixture to cook for four to five minutes.
- Top with parmesan and enjoy.

Zesty Tilapia

This recipe makes 4 servings, and contains 173 calories; 7 grams fat; 23 grams protein; 2 grams net carbohydrates per serving

What You Need

- Chopped parsley, 2 tsp.
- Pepper
- Minced garlic, 2 cloves
- Salt

- Juice of a lemon
- Lime juice, 1 tbsp.
- Melted butter, 2 tbsp.
- Tilapia, 4 fillets

What to Do

- Clean and dry the tilapia.
- Place your oven to 375.
- Combine the pepper, salt, parsley, garlic, butter, lemon juice, and lime juice together.
- Lay the tilapia in a baking dish and cover with the sauce. Bake the fish for 30 minutes. It should flake easily with a fork when done.
- Serve the fish with steamed asparagus or a salad.

Avocado Pesto Zoodles

This recipe makes 4 servings, and contains 526 calories; 49 grams fat; 12 grams protein; 6 grams net carbohydrates per serving

What You Need

Pesto

- Olive oil, 2 tbsp.
- Salt, 1 tsp.
- Pine nuts, .25 c
- Garlic, 3 cloves
- Fresh basil, 1 c
- Lemon juice, 1 tbsp.
- Avocados, 2

Pasta

- Parmesan, .5 c
- Bacon, 6 slices
- Olive oil, 1 tbsp.
- Spiralized zucchini, 4

What to Do

- Start by spiralizing your zucchini and place them on paper towels to drain.
- Add the salt, lemon juice, pine nuts, garlic, basil leaves, and avocados to your food processor. Mix for about 20-30 seconds. Add in the olive oil and mix until it creates a creamy sauce.
- Cook your bacon in a skillet until it is crispy. Lay the bacon on paper towels to dry. Once the bacon is cool enough to handle, crumble and set to the side.
- Add a tablespoon of oil to a pan. Cook the zoodles and toss them in the oil. Cook them for about two minutes or until tender.
- Add the zoodles to a bowl and pour in the pesto sauce. Toss everything together and top with the crumbled bacon and parmesan cheese. Enjoy.

Roasted Chicken with Veggies

This recipe makes 6 servings, and contains 407 calories; 28 grams fat; 23 grams protein; 11 grams net carbohydrates per serving

What You Need

- Pepper, 1 tsp.
- Rosemary, 1 tsp.
- Minced garlic, 3 cloves
- Chopped celery, 4 stalks
- Salt, 1 tsp.
- Chopped carrots, 2 small
- Medium onion sliced into wedges
- Olive oil, 3 tbsp.

- Bone-in, skin-on chicken thighs, 6

What to Do

- Start by placing your oven to 400.
- Pour the oil into a large bowl and add in the pepper, rosemary, salt, garlic, celery, carrot, and onion. Toss everything together.
- Grease a baking dish and spread the veggies in the bottom.
- Rub the chicken thighs with pepper and salt and lay on top of the veggies.
- Cook everything until the veggies are tender and the chicken is cooked and browned. This should take about 35-40 minutes.
- Allow the chicken to rest for five minutes before serving.

Shrimp Scampi with Zoodles

This recipe makes 4 servings, and contains 162 calories; 7 grams fat; 18 grams protein; 5 grams net carbohydrates per serving

What You Need

- Parsley – garnish
- Parmesan, 2 tbsp.
- Spiralized zucchini, 4
- Juice of a lemon
- Chicken stock, .25 c
- Red pepper flakes, .5 tsp.
- Minced garlic, 2 cloves
- Cleaned medium shrimp, 1 lb.
- Butter, 2 tbsp.

What to Do

- Melt the butter in a skillet. Add in the red pepper flakes and garlic. Cook everything for a minute, constantly stirring.

- Add in the shrimp and cook for around three minutes.

- Mix in the lemon juice and chicken stock.

- Mix the zoodles into the mixture and cook, occasionally stirring, for around two more minutes.

- Sprinkle with some pepper and salt.

- Serve the shrimp scampi with some parsley and parmesan.

Taco Rolls

This recipe makes 4 servings, and contains 583 calories; 40 grams fat; 48 grams protein; 3 grams net carbohydrates per serving

What You Need

- Chopped cilantro
- Tomato sauce, 1 can
- Onion powder, .5 tsp.
- Cayenne, .25 tsp.
- Cumin, .5 tsp.
- Garlic salt, .5 tsp.
- Chopped avocado, .5
- Chopped tomatoes, 25 c
- Ground beef, 1 lb.
- Taco sauce, 2 tsp.
- Cheddar cheese, 2.5 c

What to Do

- Start by heating your oven to 400.

- Heat up a large pan and add in the beef. Cook until browned. This will take around five to seven minutes.

- Season with some cumin, garlic salt, and onion powder.

- Add in the tomato sauce and stir everything together so that the meat is coated. Simmer until the mixture has thickened. This will take about five minutes.

- Lay some parchment paper in a baking sheet and spritz with cooking spray.

- Cover the baking sheet with cheddar cheese.

- Bake this for about 15 minutes. The cheese should be melted and bubbly but not burnt.

- Take out of the oven and top with the taco meat. Bake for six to eight minutes more.

- Take this out of the oven and carefully hold the sides of the parchment to remove from the baking sheet.

- Top with the cilantro, avocados, and tomatoes.

- With a pizza cutter, slice it from top to bottom into four slices.

- Carefully roll them up to make the taco rolls. Serve with a salad.

Fajita Bowl

This recipe makes 4 servings, and contains 402 calories; 22 grams fat; 33 grams protein; 13 grams net carbohydrates per serving

What You Need

Fajita Seasoning

- Cumin, .25 tsp.
- Oregano, 1 tsp.
- Garlic powder, .25 tsp.
- Salt, .5 tsp.
- Chili powder, .5 tsp.
- Paprika, .5 tsp.

Fajitas

- Chopped cilantro, .5 c
- Sour cream, 8 oz.
- Jalapenos, .5 c
- Cherry tomatoes, 1 c
- Cubed avocado, 1 c
- Lettuce, 2 c
- Juice of ½ lime
- Sliced yellow bell pepper
- Chicken broth, .25 c
- Olive oil, 2 tbsp.
- Sliced medium onion
- Sliced red bell pepper

What to Do

- Mix all of the fajita seasoning ingredients together.
- Add two tablespoons of oil to a skillet and heat. Once hot, mix in the chicken and cook five to seven minutes, or until cooked and golden.
- Mix in the bell peppers, onion, and fajita seasoning. Let this cook for another four to five minutes, or until everything is tender.
- Mix in the chicken brother and lime juice and let it start to boil. Turn the heat down, and cook for ten minutes.
- Place lettuce in a serving bowl and add in the fajita meat and veggies, avocado, tomatoes, jalapenos, sour cream, and then cilantro. Enjoy.

Portobello Pizza

This recipe makes 4 servings, and contains 251 calories; 20 grams fat; 14 grams protein; 4 grams net carbohydrates per serving

What You Need

- Shredded mozzarella, 1 c

- Chopped basil, 2 tsp.
- Sliced tomato, 1
- Minced garlic, 1 tsp.
- Olive oil, .25 c
- Portobello mushrooms, 4 large

What to Do

- You need to warm your oven to broil.
- Place aluminum foil onto a baking sheet. Grease the mushrooms with olive oil gently so you don't break them.
- Put the mushrooms onto the baking sheet with the gill side down.
- Place into the oven for two minutes.
- Turn them over and broil for one more minute.
- Remove from oven and evenly spread the garlic over each.
- Top with a slice of tomato, a sprinkle of basil, and top with cheese.
- Broil the mushrooms once more until cheese is bubbly and melted.

Carbonara

This recipe makes 4 servings, and contains 453 calories; 80 grams fat; 25 grams protein; 9 grams net carbohydrates per serving

What You Need

- Chopped parsley
- Pepper
- Salt
- Egg yolks, 4
- Heavy whipping cream, 1.25 c
- Mayonnaise, .25 c

- Butter, 1 tbsp.
- Zucchini, 2
- Sliced bacon, 8

What to Do

- Place the cream in a pot and allow to boil. Turn the heat down and continue cooking for a few minutes until reduced by a fourth.
- Cook the bacon until crisp. Keep the fat to be used later.
- Add the mayonnaise to the cream and season with pepper and salt. Let this cook until warmed through.
- Use a spiralizer to turn the zucchini into noodles. You could also make strips with a vegetable peeler.
- Put the "zoodles" into the cream sauce. Divide these out into four bowls and top with parmesan, bacon, parsley, and the egg yolks. Toss to combine.
- Drizzle with bacon grease and enjoy.

Pizza

This recipe makes 2 servings, and contains 459 calories; 90 grams fat; 55 grams protein; 8 grams net carbohydrates per serving

What You Need

- Oregano, 1 tsp.
- Shredded cheddar, 5 oz.
- Olives
- Eggs, 4
- Pepperoni, 1.5 oz.
- Tomato paste, 3 tbsp.
- Shredded cheddar, 6 oz.

What to Do

- You need to warm your oven to 400.

- Crack the eggs in a bowl and add in six ounces of cheese. Stir until they are well combined.

- Place parchment paper onto a baking sheet and spread the cheese batter into a thin crust. You could make two round crusts if you wanted to. Bake for 15 minutes. Take out of the oven and allow to cool.

- Raise the oven temp to 450.

- Spread the tomato paste on top of the crust and sprinkle with oregano. Add the remaining cheese, pepperoni, and olives.

- Bake again for ten minutes. Serve with a salad.

Thai Zoodles

This recipe makes 2 servings, and contains 644 calories; 39 grams fat; 47 grams protein; 12 grams net carbohydrates per serving

What You Need

Zoodles

- Chopped cilantro, .25 c
- Crushed peanuts, .33 c
- Bean sprouts, 1 c
- Coconut oil, 1.5 tbsp.
- Chopped green onion, .5 c
- Eggs, 2
- Shrimp, 7 oz.
- Spiralized zucchini, 2
- Lime wedges

Dressing

- Juice of a lime

- Soy sauce, 3 tbsp.
- Liquid stevia, 7 drops
- Fish sauce, 1 tbsp.
- Water, .25 c
- Peanut butter, 2 tbsp.

What to Do

- Start out by spiralizing the zucchini and set the zoodles on some paper towels to drain.
- Mix all of the dressing ingredients together.
- Add in ½ tablespoon of coconut oil to a large skillet and scramble the eggs and then set them to the side.
- Mix in the shrimp to the same pan and cook until the shrimp is pink and cooked through about three minutes. Set the shrimp to the side.
- Add a tablespoon of coconut oil in the pan and mix in the zoodles. Cook them until tender, two to three minutes.
- Add in the cooked shrimp, scrambled eggs, and green onions.
- Pour in the sauce and cook for another minute. Mix in the bean sprouts.
- Serve the Pad Thai topped with a lime wedge, cilantro, and crushed peanuts.

Ricotta and Spinach Gnocchi

This recipe makes 4 servings, and contains 125 calories; 8 grams fat; 6 grams protein; 4 grams net carbohydrates per serving

What You Need

- Butter, 2 tbsp.
- Water, 2.5 c
- Almond flour, just encase
- Pepper
- Salt

- Egg
- Nutmeg, .25 tsp.
- Ricotta, 1 c
- Chopped frozen spinach, 3 c

What to Do

- Place the spinach on a paper towel or cheesecloth and squeeze the excess liquid from it. Place it in a bowl.
- Add pepper, salt, nutmeg, egg, half of the parmesan, and the ricotta cheese into the same bowl. Mix all of the ingredients together so that they are all well combined.
- Allow a large pot to come to a boil. Scoop out tablespoon size of the spinach mixture and roll into a cylinder shape. For a traditional gnocchi look, roll a fork across it to create lines. Add this first gnocchi to the boiling water, if the gnocchi breaks apart, mix in some almond flour to the rest of your mixture. Repeat this until the gnocchi holds together in the water.
- Once the gnocchi holds together, form the rest of the spinach mixture into the gnocchi rounds and cook them in the boiling water. Once they rise to the top of the water, they are done. This will take about two minutes. Take the gnocchi out with a perforated spoon.
- Melt the butter and serve the gnocchi with the melted butter over top. Sprinkle on some parmesan cheese and serve with a salad.

Dinner

Turkey Meatloaf

This recipe makes 6 servings, and contains 216 calories; 19 grams fat; 15 grams protein; 1 gram net carbohydrates per serving

What You Need

- Pepper
- Salt
- Chopped parsley, 1 tbsp.
- Parmesan, .25 c
- Heavy cream, .33 c
- Ground turkey, 1.5 lbs.
- Chopped onion, .5
- Olive oil, 1 tbsp.

What to Do

- Start by placing your oven to 450.
- Pour the olive oil to a skillet and cook the onion until tender, about four minutes.
- Place the onion in a bowl and stir in the pepper, parsley, salt, parmesan, heavy cream, and turkey. Make sure everything is very well combined. Using your hands works better than a spoon to make sure everything is well combined.
- Press the meat into a loaf pan.
- Bake for 30 minutes.
- Allow the meatloaf to rest for ten before serving.

Haddock

This recipe makes 4 servings, and contains 299 calories; 24 grams fat; 20 grams protein; 1 gram net carbohydrates per serving

What You Need

- Melted coconut oil, 2 tbsp.
- Ground hazelnuts, .25 c
- Shredded unsweetened coconut, 1 c
- Pepper
- Salt
- Boneless haddock 4 5-oz. fillets

What to Do

- Start by placing your oven to 400. Place parchment paper on a baking sheet.
- Dry off the fillets with a paper towel and then sprinkle them with pepper and salt on both sides.
- Mix the hazelnuts and shredded coconut together.
- Brush the fillets with coconut oil and then press the coconut mixture into the fish.
- Bake the fish for 12 minutes. It should flake apart easily. Serve.

Zucchini Gratin

This recipe makes 4 servings, and contains 371 calories; 33 grams fat; 13 grams protein; 4 grams net carbohydrates per serving

What You Need

- Pepper
- Salt
- Shredded cheese, 1.5 c

- Heavy cream, 1 c
- Sliced yellow squash, 2
- Sliced zucchini, 2
- Minced garlic, 2 cloves
- Diced small onion
- Butter, 2 tbsp.

What to Do

- Start by placing your oven to 350.
- Melt the butter in a skillet. Mix in the onions and cook until they become translucent.
- Mix in the garlic and sauté everything for a minute.
- Mix in the heavy cream and a cup of the cheese. Make sure you stir quickly and make sure everything is well mixed, and cheese has melted.
- Let the sauce simmer until it has thickened.
- Meanwhile, grease a baking dish with some cooking spray.
- Lay the squash and zucchini in the baking dish. Pour the cheese sauce on the veggies and top with the remaining shredded cheese.
- Bake this for 30 minutes, or until it has thickened and the top has browned.
- Serve.

Cauliflower Mac and Cheese

This recipe makes 4 servings, and contains 434 calories; 39 grams fat; 15 grams protein; 5 grams net carbohydrates per serving

What You Need

- Pepper
- Salt
- Garlic powder, .5 tsp.
- Dijon, 1 tsp.

- Shredded cheddar, 1 ½ c – divided
- Cubed cream cheese, 4 oz.
- Heavy cream, .5 c
- Olive oil, 2 tsp.
- Butter, 2 tbsp.
- Bacon, 2 slices
- Cauliflower, 1 head – cut into florets

What to Do

- Start by setting your oven to 425 and heat the oil in a pan.
- Place the cauliflower and bacon to the pan and cook for five minutes.
- Pour this into a casserole dish and place this to the side.
- In a pot, add a cup of the cheddar, and the heavy cream, Dijon, and butter. Cook, stirring until everything is melted and combined. Whisk the cream cheese into the mixture until melted and smooth. Season with the garlic powder, pepper, and salt.
- Pour the cheese over the cauliflower and mix everything together. Sprinkle on the remaining cheese and bake for 15 minutes. The top should be browned. Enjoy.

Lettuce Wrap Cheeseburger

This recipe makes 1 serving, and contains 601 calories; 51 grams fat; 26 grams protein; 5 grams net carbohydrates per serving

What You Need

- Mayonnaise, 1 tsp.
- Oregano, 1 tsp.
- Salt, .5 tsp.
- Onion, 3 rings
- Pepper, .25 tsp.
- Lettuce leaves

- Slice cheese
- Ground beef, 5 oz.

What to Do

- Season the meat with oregano, pepper, and salt. Form the meat into a patty.
- Grill the burger for four to five minutes on both sides, or until it is cooked to your liking.
- Once the burger is cooked, take it off the grill and top with a slice of cheese and lay it on top of the lettuce leaf.
- Top with the onion and mayonnaise. Wrap the lettuce around and enjoy.

Pork Loin with Mustard Sauce

This recipe makes 8 servings, and contains 368 calories; 29 grams fat; 25 grams protein; 2 grams net carbohydrates per serving

What You Need

- Grainy mustard, 3 tbsp.
- Heavy cream, 1.5 c
- Olive oil, 3 tbsp.
- Pepper
- Salt
- Boneless pork loin roast, 2 lb.

What to Do

- Start by placing your oven to 375.
- Rub the pork loin with pepper and salt.
- Heat the oil in a large skillet. Place the roast in the hot pan and sear on all sides. Lay in a baking dish.
- Finish cooking the roast in the oven for an hour.

- When about 15 minutes remain on the roasting time, add the mustard and heavy cream to a pot. Stir together and allow it to start boiling. Lower to a simmer and allow the mixture to continue to simmer until it has thickened up about five minutes. Set it off the heat.
- Once the pork is cooked to your liking, allow it to cool for ten minutes before slicing. Serve with a drizzle of the mustard sauce.

Lamb with Sun-Dried Tomatoes

This recipe makes 8 servings, and contains 352 calories; 29 grams fat; 17 grams protein; 3 grams net carbohydrates per serving

What You Need

Lamb

- Olive oil, 2 tbsp.
- Pepper
- Salt
- Boneless lamb leg, 2 lb.

Pesto

- Minced garlic, 2 tsp.
- Chopped basil, 2 tbsp.
- EVOO, 2 tbsp.
- Pine nuts, .25 c
- Sun-dried tomatoes, 1 c

What to Do

- ***For the pesto*** – Place the pest ingredients to your food processor and mix until the sauce becomes smooth. Set aside.
- ***For the lamb*** – begin by placing your oven to 400.
- Rub the leg of lamb with pepper and salt.

- Add the oil to an ovenproof skillet and heat. Sear the lamb on all sides until it has browned up.

- Rub the leg of lamb with the pesto sauce. Roast for an hour, or until the lamb has reached your desired doneness.

- Allow the lamb to sit for ten minutes before slicing and serving.

Thai Lettuce Wrap

This recipe makes 6 servings, and contains 286 calories; 15 grams fat; 22 grams protein; 13 grams net carbohydrates per serving

What You Need

- Pepper
- Salt
- Chopped peanuts, .25 c
- Chopped cilantro, .25 c
- Chopped green onions, 3
- Chopped large onion
- Minced garlic, 3 cloves
- Diced chicken breasts, 1 lb.
- Olive oil, 1 tbsp.
- Large head iceberg

Sauce

- Ginger, .25 tsp.
- Peanut butter, 1 tbsp.
- Chili sauce, .25 c
- Soy sauce, 1 tbsp.
- Juice of ½ lime

- Fish sauce, 2 tsp.

What to Do

- Heat the oil in a large skillet.
- Add in the onion, stir often, cooking until soft. This will take about four minutes.
- Stir in the garlic, cooking for another minute.
- Mix in the chicken and turn the heat up. Cook for about three minutes, or until the chicken is almost cooked.
- Add the sauce ingredients to a bowl and mix them together.
- Pour the sauce into the skillet with the chicken and stir everything to coat. Continue the cook until the chicken is cooked all the way through. This will take about five minutes more.
- Mix in the peanuts, cilantro, and green onions. Toss everything together. Taste, and adjust any seasonings that you need to.
- Spoon the chicken into the lettuce leaves and serve.

Cheeseburger

This recipe makes 4 servings, and contains 850 calories; 67 grams fat; 49 grams protein; 7 grams net carbohydrates per serving

What You Need

- Pepper, .5 tsp.
- Salt, 1 tsp.
- Peanut butter, 4 tbsp.
- Bacon, 20 slices
- Onion powder, 1 tsp.
- Cheddar cheese, 2 oz.
- Garlic powder, 1 tsp.
- Ground beef, 1 lb.

What to Do

- Using your hands, mix together the ground beef and the seasonings. Form the meat into four patties.

- Grill the burgers until they are almost done. They will cook more, later on, so you don't want them to become tough.

- Once the burgers are done, spread each with a tablespoon of peanut butter and top with a sprinkle of cheese.

- Wrap five slices of bacon around each burger and lay them on a cookie sheet.

- Cook the burgers for 20 minutes at 400. Cook until the bacon is done to your liking.

- Serve your burger with onion, lettuce, and any other desired toppings.

Tri-Tip

This recipe makes 4 servings, and contains 693 calories; 44 grams fat; 68 grams protein; 0 gram net carbohydrates per serving

What You Need

- Salt, .5 tbsp.
- Pepper, 1 tsp.
- Minced garlic clove
- Olive oil, 3 tbsp.
- Tri-tip steak, 2 lbs.

What to Do

- Mix together the pepper, salt, oil, and garlic. Rub the steak with the marinade and refrigerate it for a couple of hours.

- Heat up a skillet and place in the steak. Cook the steak for five minutes on both sides.

- Slice the steak and serve with a salad.

Sausage Casserole

This recipe makes 4 servings, and contains 332 calories; 26 grams fat; 18 grams protein; 4

grams net carbohydrates per serving

What You Need

- Shredded cheddar, 1 c
- Ground sage, 1 tsp.
- Mayonnaise, 2 tsp.
- Eggs, 3
- Diced zucchini, 2
- Dijon, 1 tsp.
- Diced onion, .5 c
- Pork sausage, .5 lb.

What to Do

- Start by placing your oven to 375.
- Grease a baking dish with some nonstick spray.
- Heat up a large pan and add in the sausage. Cook until the sausage has browned up, about two minutes.
- Mix in the onion and zucchini. Cook for another four to five minutes or until the veggies become tender.
- Spoon this into the greased baking dish.
- Stir together ½ cup of cheese, the sage, mustard, mayonnaise, and eggs.
- Pour this over the sausage mixture.
- Top with the rest of the cheese and bake for 25 minutes. Enjoy.

Sausage Crust Pizza

This recipe makes 4 servings, and contains 357 calories; 21 grams fat; 31 grams protein; 12 grams net carbohydrates per serving

What You Need

- Italian seasoning, 1 tsp.
- Onion powder, 1 tsp.
- Tomato paste, 1 tbsp.
- Sliced ham, 2 oz.
- Garlic powder, 1 tsp.
- Diced red bell pepper
- Diced and sautéed small onion
- Mozzarella cheese, 3 oz.
- Sautéed mushrooms, 2 oz.
- Sausage, 1 lb.

What to Do

- Start by placing your oven to 350.
- Mash the sausage into the bottom and sides of a medium cake pan. Bake this for 10-15 minutes.
- Take the crust out and drain off any grease that has accumulated.
- Combine the Italian seasoning, onion powder, garlic powder, and tomato paste. Spread this over the crust.
- Top with the mushrooms, bell pepper, ham, and onions.
- Sprinkle the top with the mozzarella.
- Cook the pizza until the cheese is melted and bubbly, about 12-15 minutes.

Garlic Parmesan Salmon

This recipe makes 2 servings, and contains 480 calories; 33 grams fat; 35 grams protein; 8 grams net carbohydrates per serving

What You Need

- Pepper

- Salt
- Chopped parsley, 1 bunch
- Heavy cream, .25 c
- Parmesan, .5 c
- Minced garlic, 3 cloves
- Butter, 2 tbsp.
- Salmon, 2 9-oz. fillets

What to Do

- Start by placing your oven to 350.
- Line a baking sheet with parchment.
- Lay the salmon on the baking sheet and sprinkle with some pepper and salt and set to the side.
- Melt the butter in a skillet. Mix in the garlic and sauté until softened. Turn the heat down and mix in the parmesan and heavy cream. Mix everything together until melted.
- Pour this over the salmon.
- Bake for 15-20 minutes. Sprinkle on a little more salt and top with some parsley. Serve with a salad.

Coconut Lime Skirt Steak

This recipe makes 3 servings, and contains 787 calories; 48 grams fat; 89 grams protein; 2 grams net carbohydrates per serving

What You Need

- Salt, 1 tsp.
- Grated ginger, 1 tbsp.
- Lime juice, 2 tbsp.
- Melted coconut oil, .5 c
- Minced garlic, 1 tbsp.

- Skirt steak, 2 lbs.

What to Do

- Combine the salt, ginger, garlic, lime juice, and melted coconut oil together.
- Add the steak in a bag and add in the marinade. Allow this to sit for at least 30 minutes. Make sure you don't skip this.
- Grill the steak for at least four minutes on each side. You can cook it longer to reach your desired level of doneness. Slice and serve.

Creamy Butter Chicken

This recipe makes 6 servings, and contains 319 calories; 20 grams fat; 26 grams protein; 5 grams net carbohydrates per serving

What You Need

For Serving

- Cooked cauliflower rice
- Chopped cilantro

Sauce

- Garam masala, .5 tbsp.
- Heavy cream, .5 c
- Cumin, 1 tsp.
- Chili powder, 1 tsp.
- Crushed tomatoes, small can
- Minced garlic, 2 tsp.
- Tomato paste, 2 tbsp.
- Grated ginger, 2 tsp.
- Chopped onion

- Ghee, 2 tbsp.
- Chicken –
- Plain yogurt, 4 oz.
- Minced garlic, 3 cloves
- Olive oil, 1 tbsp.
- Grated ginger, 3 tsp.
- Garam masala, 2 tbsp.

Diced chicken breast, 1.5 lbs.

What to Do

- Add the chicken and two tablespoons of garam masala, along with the yogurt, minced garlic, and grated ginger to a bowl and mix them together. Chill the chicken for at least 20 minutes.
- For the sauce – add the tomato paste, tomatoes, garlic, ginger, and onion to a blender and combine everything until smooth. Set to the side.
- Heat a tablespoon of oil in a large pan.
- Add the chicken to the pan and sauté for four to five minutes, or until it turns golden.
- Add the sauce into the chicken and cook for another four to six minutes more.
- Mix in the ghee and heavy cream. Turn the heat down and cook for another five minutes.
- Serve the chicken over top of the cooked cauliflower rice and topped with cilantro.

Buffalo Chicken

This recipe makes 2 servings, and contains 685 calories; 43 grams fat; 57 grams protein; 12 grams net carbohydrates per serving

What You Need

- Pepper, 2 tsp.
- Chili powder, 1 tsp.
- Garlic powder, 1 tsp.

- Eggs, 2
- Salt, 2 tsp.
- Blue cheese dip, .5 c
- Butter, 2 tbsp.
- Hot sauce, .25 c
- Paprika, 1 tsp.
- Almond flour, 2 tbsp.
- Chicken breast strips, 1 lb.

What to Do

- Start by placing your oven to 400.
- Line a baking sheet with parchment.
- Mix together the pepper, salt, chili powder, paprika, and garlic powder.
- Rub a quarter of the spice mixture onto the chicken.
- Place the remaining seasonings to the almond flour and mix together.
- Beat the eggs together in a separate bowl.
- Coat the chicken tender in the egg and then dip into the almond flour. Lay the chicken on your baking sheet. Repeat this for the rest of the chicken.
- Bake the chicken tenders for 25 minutes. They should reach 165.
- Meanwhile, add the butter to a pot and melt. Mix in the hot sauce and combined well.
- Once the chicken is done, drizzle the hot sauce over the chicken. You can also toss the chicken tenders in the sauce to completely cover them.
- Serve with the blue cheese dip.

Sausage and Veggies

This recipe makes 4 servings, and contains 220 calories; 12 grams fat; 15 grams protein; 10 grams net carbohydrates per serving

What You Need

- Pepper
- Salt
- Italian seasoning, .5 tsp.
- Vegetable broth, .5 c
- Baby spinach, 1 c
- Medium zucchini sliced into half-moon shapes
- Chopped yellow bell pepper
- Chopped mushrooms, 1 c
- Chopped red bell pepper
- Sliced onion
- Minced garlic, 2 cloves
- Cooked, sliced Italian chicken sausage, 12 oz.
- Olive oil, 1.5 tbsp.

What to Do

- Heat the oil in a large pan.
- Mix in the onion and sausage and cook until the onions have become tender.
- Mix in the garlic, cooking everything for another minute.
- Mix in the pepper, salt, Italian seasoning, mushrooms, bell peppers, and zucchini. Sauté everything for two minutes.
- Pour in the broth and let the mixture come to a boil. Lower to a simmer and cook for ten minutes.
- Mix in the spinach, cooking until wilted.
- Serve.

Stuffed Peppers

This recipe makes 2 servings, and contains 453 calories; 30 grams fat; 28 grams protein; 9 grams net carbohydrates per serving

What You Need

- Pepper
- Salt
- Shredded cheddar, .25 c
- Chopped cilantro, .25 c
- Sliced mushrooms, 8
- Minced garlic clove
- Poblano peppers halved vertically, 4
- Coconut oil, 1 tbsp.
- Chorizo sausage, .5 lb.

What to Do

- Start by placing the oven to 375.
- Let the peppers on a baking sheet and slide them in the oven for ten minutes.
- Meanwhile, add the chorizo in a skillet with the coconut oil and cook for four to five minutes, or until browned.
- Mix in the garlic, stirring until fragrant. Mix in the mushrooms.
- After the mushrooms have browned up, mix in the cilantro and cook for three minutes more.
- Take the peppers out of the oven and divide the chorizo mixture between them. Sprinkle the tops of the peppers with the cheddar.
- Cook the peppers for eight minutes.
- Serve.

Crispy Wings

This recipe makes 2 servings, and contains 582 calories; 16 grams fat; 99 grams protein; 5 grams net carbohydrates per serving

What You Need

- Salt, 2 tsp.
- Chicken wings, 2 lbs.
- Baking powder, 1.5 tbsp.

What to Do

- Set your oven to 250.
- Get the chicken wings as dry as possible and then lay them in a plastic bag. Pour in the salt and baking powder. Shake everything together so that they are well coated.
- Spread the chicken wings out on a baking sheet and slide them in the oven for 30 minutes.
- Turn the temperature up to 425 and continue to cook the chicken for 20-30 minutes, or until they are completely cooked.
- You can enjoy them as is or toss them in your favorite sauce.

Pulled Pork

This recipe makes 8 servings, and contains 464 calories; 30 grams fat; 43 grams protein; 2 grams net carbohydrates per serving

What You Need

- Bay leaves, 3
- Garlic powder, 2 tsp.
- Salt, 3 tsp.
- Boneless pork shoulder, 3 lb.
- Paprika, 1 tsp.
- Chopped onion

What to Do

- Flip your crock pot to low.

- Combine some salt, paprika, and garlic powder.

- Slice some lines into the surface of the pork should so that it has some areas to catch the spices. Rub the spice mixture into the pork.

- Lay the pork and the onion into your crock pot.

- Top with the bay leaves.

- Place on the lid and let it cook for ten minutes.

- Once it's cooked through, remove the bay leaves, and shred the pork.

- Serve hot with your favorite low-carb barbecue sauce.

Dijon Chicken with Vegetables

This recipe makes 4 servings, and contains 603 calories; 46 grams fat; 34 grams protein; 8 grams net carbohydrates per serving

What You Need

- Juice of lemon
- Cauliflower florets, 2 c
- Broccoli florets, 2 c
- Medium carrots cut into 4-inch pieces, 4
- Fresh thyme, 1 tbsp.
- Minced garlic clove
- Dijon, 3 tbsp. – divided
- Sliced medium onion, 3
- Olive oil, 4 tbsp. – divided
- Salt, 3 tsp. – divided
- Skin-on bone-in chicken thighs, 4

What to Do

- Start by placing your oven to 425.

- Mix together two teaspoons of salt, a tablespoon of garlic, two tablespoons of mustard, and two tablespoons of oil. Brush the mixture onto the chicken thighs.

- Lay the chicken thighs with the skin side up on a baking sheet. Bake the chicken for ten minutes.

- As the chicken is cooking, mix together the rest of the salt, oil, and mustard, along with the lemon juice, and thyme. Toss in the cauliflower, broccoli, carrots, and onions. Toss everything together.

- Lay the vegetables on a baking sheet. Once ten minutes of cooking time has passed, add the veggies to the oven and let everything cook for 25 minutes more, or until the chicken is cooked and the vegetables are tender.

- Garnish with some extra thyme.

Indian-Style Chicken

This recipe makes 4 servings, and contains 563 calories; 30 grams fat; 63 grams protein; 4 grams net carbohydrates per serving

What You Need

- Pepper
- Salt
- Steamed broccoli, 4 c
- Cumin, 1 tsp.
- Full-fat Greek yogurt, 1 c
- Chopped onion
- Turmeric, .5 tsp.
- Grated ginger, 1 tbsp.
- Olive oil, 1 tbsp.
- Cayenne, .5 tsp.
- Minced garlic, 3 cloves
- Boneless, skinless chicken breasts, 4

What to Do

- Add the pepper, salt, turmeric, cayenne, oil, ginger, onion, yogurt, and chicken to a plastic bag and toss everything together.

- Refrigerate the chicken for at least two hours.

- Set your oven to 350.

- Grease a baking sheet.

- Take the chicken out of the bag and lay it out on the baking sheet. Cook the chicken for ten minutes.

- Take the chicken out of the oven and flip. Cook for another ten minutes.

- Slice the chicken and serve with the steamed broccoli.

Mexican Meatloaf

This recipe makes 8 servings, and contains 372 calories; 20 grams fat; 40 grams protein; 2 grams net carbohydrates per serving

What You Need

- Chopped small onion

- Grated cheddar, 1 c

- Chili powder, 2 tsp.

- Pork rind crumbs, 1 c

- Pepper, .5 tsp.

- Cumin, 2 tsp.

- Salsa, .5 c

- Eggs, 2

- Ground beef, 2 lbs.

What to Do

- Start by placing your oven to 350.

- Mix together the onion, pepper, cumin, chili powder, eggs, pork rinds, and ground beef. Using your hands is the best option because you can get everything mixed together better.

- Press half of the meatloaf mixture into a loaf pan.

- Sprinkle half of a cup of the cheese.

- Press the rest of the meatloaf mixture over top of the cheese.

- Bake the meatloaf for an hour.

- Top with the remaining cheese and bake for an additional ten minutes, or until the cheese has melted.

- Allow the meatloaf to rest for ten minutes before slicing and serving.

Chicken Enchiladas

This recipe makes 4 servings, and contains 297 calories; 16 grams fat; 32 grams protein; 3 grams net carbohydrates per serving

What You Need

- Shredded cheddar, 1 c
- Shredded Jack cheese, 1 c
- Cumin, 2 tsp.
- Chili powder, 2 tsp.
- Butter, 1 tbsp.
- Zucchinis sliced into flat sheets, 4
- Cubed medium onion
- Shredded cooked chicken, 1 lb.

Enchilada Sauce

- Pepper, 1 tsp.
- Onion powder, 1 tsp.
- Hot sauce, .5 tsp.

- Garlic powder, 1 tsp.
- Water, .5 c
- Olive oil, .25 c
- Italian seasoning, 1 tsp.
- Tomato paste, 1 can

What to Do

- Start by placing your oven to 350.
- Mix all of the sauce ingredients together.
- Melt the butter in a large skillet. Sauté the onions in the butter until they are soft, about three to four minutes.
- Mix in the cumin, chili powder, shredded chicken, and a cup of the enchilada sauce. Set to the side.
- Lay four slices of zucchini side by side, overlapping them slightly.
- Add a spoonful of the chicken to one end of the zucchini and roll them up. Place it in the casserole dish.
- Continue this process until you have used the rest of the chicken and zucchini.
- Next, pour the rest of the enchilada sauce over the rolled zucchini and then sprinkle both kinds of cheese over the top.
- Slide them in the oven and cook for 20 to 25 minutes, or until the cheese has melted and is bubbly.
- Serve with any of your favorite toppings like sour cream.

Halibut Butter Sauce

This recipe makes 4 servings, and contains 319 calories; 26 grams fat; 22 grams protein; 2 grams net carbohydrates per serving

What You Need

- Olive oil, 2 tbsp.
- Halibut fillets, 4 5-oz. fillets

- Pepper
- Chopped parsley, 1 tsp.
- Lemon juice, 1 tbsp.
- Butter, .25 c
- Orange juice, 1 tbsp.
- Minced garlic, 2 tsp.
- Minced shallot
- Dry white wine, 3 tbsp.

What to Do

- Pat the halibut dry so that it holds onto the seasoning. Rub the pepper and salt into the fish. Lay on a plate lined with paper towels and set to the side.
- Place the butter to a pot and allow it to melt.
- Add in the garlic and shallot and cook until it becomes tender. This will take around three minutes.
- Mix in the orange juice, white wine, and lemon juice. Allow this sauce to simmer and cook until it has slightly thickened. This is going to take around two minutes.
- Set it off the heat and mix in the parsley. Set to the side.
- Heat up a large skillet with the olive oil.
- Fry up the fish until it is golden and cooked all the way through, flipping only once. This will take around ten minutes.
- Serve the fish with a spoonful of the butter sauce.

Lamb Chops with Tapenade

This recipe makes 4 servings, and contains 348 calories; 28 grams fat; 21 grams protein; 1 gram net carbohydrates per serving

What You Need

Tapenade

- Chopped fresh parsley, 2 tbsp.
- Kalamata olives, 1 c
- Lemon juice, 2 tsp.
- Minced garlic, 2 tsp.
- EVOO, 2 tbsp.

Lamb Chops

- French-cut lamb chips, 2 1-lb. racks
- Olive oil, 1 tbsp.
- Pepper
- Salt

What to Do

- To make the tapenade, place the olives, lemon juice, parsley, garlic, and olive oil in a food processor and mix until it is completely pureed, but still a little bit chunky.
- Pour the tapenade into a container and keep it refrigerated until you need it.
- To make the lamb chops, start by setting your oven to 450. Rub the pepper and the salt into the lamb.
- Drizzle the oil into an ovenproof skillet and allow it to heat up. Lay the lamb racks in the pan and sear on all sides.
- Sit the racks upright in the heated pan. The bones need to be interlaced. Roast the lamb in the oven until it has reached your desired level of doneness. 20 minutes will bring the lamb to about medium-rare. At the very least it should reach 125.
- Once the lamb is finished cooking, let it rest of ten minutes. Slice up the rack of lambs into individual chops. Each person should get four chops and top each of them with some of the tapenade that you fixed earlier.

Sirloin and Butter

This recipe makes 4 servings, and contains 544 calories; 44 grams fat; 35 grams protein; 0 gram net carbohydrates per serving

What You Need

- Room temperature butter, 6 tbsp.
- Pepper
- Blue cheese, 4 oz.
- Salt
- Sirloin steaks, 4 5-oz. steaks
- Olive oil, 1 tbsp.

What to Do

- Place the butter in a blender and whip it up. This will take about two minutes.
- Place the cheese in with the butter and pulse a few times until mixed.
- Spoon the butter out on saran wrap and roll it up into a log that is about 1.5 inches in diameter.
- Refrigerate the butter for at least an hour to allow it to set up.
- Slice the butter into half-inch disks and lay them on a plate. Keep them in the refrigerator until you are ready to use them. Any leftover butter should be kept in the fridge as well, and it should last for up to a week.
- Heat a grill or skillet up. Make sure that the steak comes to room temperature before cooking.
- Rub the salt, oil, and pepper into the steaks.
- Cook the steaks until they are done to how you like them. Six minutes on both sides will bring it to medium. Remember, the steaks will continue to cook once you take them off the heat. Typically, it will rise five degrees during the resting period.
- Let the steak rest for ten minutes. Serve each steak with one of the butter disks.

Like what you're reading? Want to hear this as an audio book? Click here to get this book for FREE when you join Audible!!

https://adbl.co/2Zcx8Hq

Noodles with Beef Stroganoff Meatballs

This recipe makes 3 servings, and contains 492 calories; 39 grams fat; 19 grams protein; 14 grams net carbohydrates per serving

What You Need

- Onion powder, .5 tsp.
- Dried parsley, .5 tsp.
- Worcestershire sauce, 1 tsp.
- Almond flour, 3 tbsp.
- Pepper, .25 tsp.
- Salt, 1 tsp.
- Garlic powder, .5 tsp.
- Egg
- Ground beef, .5 tsp.

Sauce

- Butter, 2 tbsp.
- Konjac noodles, 2 servings
- Sliced mushrooms, 8 oz.
- Xanthan gum, pinch
- Sliced medium onion
- Pepper, .25 tsp.
- Minced garlic, 3 cloves
- Salt, 1 tsp.
- Beef broth, .75 c
- Sour cream, .33 c

What to Do

- Start by placing your oven to 400. Place some parchment on a cookie sheet.

- Add all of the meatball ingredients in a bowl and combine. Use an ice cream scoop to help you shape the meat into balls. Lay them on your cookie sheet and bake the meatballs for ten minutes.

- As the meatballs are cooking, add the butter to a skillet and melt. Mix in the onions, cooking until translucent. Mix in the mushrooms and cook for another seven minutes. Stir in the garlic and cook until fragrant.

- Stir in the sour cream, salt, pepper, xanthan gum, and broth. Let this mixture come up to a simmer.

- Once the meatballs have cooked in the oven, nestle them into the sauce. Cover the skillet with a lid and let everything cook together for 20 minutes.

- Top the konjac noodles with the meatballs and sauce.

Chicken Cordon Bleu Casserole

This recipe makes 4 servings, and contains 574 calories; 34 grams fat; 59 grams protein; 3 grams net carbohydrates per serving

What You Need

- Diced onion, .25 c

- Minced garlic, 2 cloves

- Dijon, 2 tsp.

- Sliced Swiss cheese, 3 oz.

- Lemon juice, 3 tbsp.

- Sliced chicken, 1 lb.

- Melted butter, .25 c + 1 tbsp.

- Sliced ham, 3 oz.

- Salt, 1 tsp.

- Softened cream cheese, 3 oz.

What to Do

- Start by placing your oven to 350. Spray a 9-inch square casserole dish with nonstick spray and set to the side.

- Add a tablespoon of butter and the diced onion to a skillet and cook until the onions become translucent. This will take about five minutes. Mix in the garlic, and cook until the garlic has become fragrant.

- Add the rest of the butter, cream cheese, Dijon, lemon juice, and salt to a blender and mix until smooth.

- Lay the chicken in your casserole dish and then add in with the onion mixture. Lay the ham over top and then spread the sauce over everything.

- Top the casserole with the sliced Swiss cheese. Bake the casserole for 35 minutes.

- Once the cooking time has ended, flip the oven to broil and bake the casserole for another two minutes until the cheese has browned and everything is bubbly. Allow the casserole to rest for a few minutes before serving.

Turkey Mushroom Bake

This recipe makes 8 servings, and contains 245 calories; 15 grams fat; 25 grams protein; 3 grams net carbohydrates per serving

What You Need

- Garlic powder, .25 tsp.
- Pepper
- Salt
- Grated parmesan, .5 c
- Grated cheddar cheese, 2 c
- Poultry seasoning, 1 tsp.
- Cream cheese, .5 c
- Chicken stock, .5 c
- Cooked and shredded turkey, 3 c
- Shredded cabbage, 3 c
- Beaten egg

- Sliced mushrooms, 4 c

What to Do

- Start by placing your oven to 375.
- Heat up a skillet and add in the salt, cream cheese, cheddar cheese, poultry seasoning, garlic powder, pepper, parmesan cheese, and egg. Mix everything together and allow it to come to a simmer.
- Mix in the turkey and cabbage and then set to the side.
- Add the mushrooms and the turkey mixture to a casserole dish and spread across the bottom.
- Cover with aluminum foil and cook the casserole for 35 minutes.
- Let the casserole rest for a few minutes before serving.

Turkey Pot Pie

This recipe makes 4 servings, and contains 325 calories; 23 grams fat; 21 grams protein; 6 grams net carbohydrates per serving

What You Need

- Cooking spray
- Xanthan gum, .25 tsp.
- Garlic powder, .25 tsp.
- Smoked paprika, .25 tsp.
- Shredded Monterey Jack, .5 c
- Chopped and peeled butternut squash, .5 c
- Chopped kale, .5 c
- Chopped fresh rosemary, 1 tsp.
- Pepper
- Salt
- Cooked and shredded turkey, 1 c

- Chicken stock, 2 c

Crust

- Cheddar cheese, .25 c
- Egg
- Pinch of salt
- Almond flour, 2 c
- Xanthan gum, .25 tsp.
- Butter, .25 c

What to Do

- Start by placing your oven to 350.
- Heat up a large pot and add in the squash and turkey. Cook the two for ten minutes. Mix in the salt, kale, smoked paprika, pepper, rosemary, garlic powder, and Monterey jack cheese.
- In a bowl, mix together the xanthan gum and stock. Pour this into the pot with everything else and mix together. Set this to the side.
- Mix the flour and xanthan gum for the crust together. Stir the rest of the crust ingredients in until it forms a dough.
- Roll into a ball and refrigerate for a few minutes while you get everything else ready.
- Grease a square baking dish with cooking spray and the turkey filling into the casserole dish.
- Take the crust out of the fridge and place it between two sheets of parchment. Roll the dough out so that it will cover the casserole dish. Lay the dough over the turkey filling and crimp down the edges to seal.
- Bake for 35 minutes.
- Allow the pie rest for a few minutes and serve.

Buttered Duck

This recipe makes 1 serving, and contains 547 calories; 46 grams fat; 35 grams protein; 2 grams net carbohydrates per serving

What You Need

- Fresh sage, .25 tsp.
- Kale, 1 c
- Pepper
- Salt
- Butter, 2 tbsp.
- Heavy cream, 1 tbsp.
- Medium duck breast – skin scored

What to Do

- Place the butter on a pan. Once melted, add in the heavy cream and the sage. Cook this for two minutes.
- In another pan, place in the duck with the skin side down. Cook the duck for four minutes to brown the skin and then flip and cook for another three minutes or until the duck is cooked through to 160.
- Add the kale to the skillet with the butter and sage. Cook this for a minute.
- Once the duck is cooked through, remove from the pan and slice. Place the duck on a plate and serve topped with the kale and butter sauce.

Cheesy Salmon

This recipe makes 4 servings, and contains 357 calories; 28 grams fat; 24 grams protein; 2 grams net carbohydrates per serving

What You Need

- Olive oil, 1 tbsp.
- Chopped basil, 1 tsp.
- Salmon filet, skin on, 4 5 oz.
- Chopped oregano, 1 tsp.
- Minced garlic, 2 tsp.

- Room temp butter, 2 tbsp.
- Lemon juice, 2 tbsp.
- Asiago cheese, .5 c

What to Do

- You need to warm your oven to 350.
- Line a baking sheet with parchment.
- Put the Asiago cheese, oregano, basil, garlic, butter, and lemon juice into a bowl. Stir together.
- Put the salmon on the prepared baking sheet with the skin down.
- Take the cheese mixture and divide it evenly between the salmon fillets. Spread it on the salmon with a spoon.
- Drizzle lightly with olive oil.
- Place in the oven for 12 minutes.

Herbed Scallops

This recipe makes 4 servings, and contains 306 calories; 24 grams fat; 19 grams protein; 4 grams net carbohydrates per serving

What You Need

- Chopped thyme, 1 tsp.
- Juice of one lemon
- Minced garlic, 2 tsp.
- Chopped basil, 2 tsp.
- Butter, 8 tbsp., divided
- Pepper
- Scallops, 1 lb.

What to Do

- Sprinkle pepper on the scallops.

- Put a large skillet on to the top of the stove and melt the butter over medium.

- Lay the scallops to the pan and sear on each side. This will take around two minutes. Take the scallops out of the skillet and place to the side.

- Put the remaining butter in the skillet and add garlic. Cook until fragrant. This takes around three minutes.

- Mix the thyme, basil and lemon juice to the garlic in the skillet. Return the scallops to the skillet.

- Spoon the butter mixture over the scallops to coat.

Buttery Lemon Chicken

This recipe makes 4 servings, and contains 294 calories; 26 grams fat; 12 grams protein; 3 grams net carbohydrates per serving

What You Need

- Juice of .5 lemon
- Heavy cream, .5 c
- Chicken stock, .5 c
- Minced garlic, 2 tsp.
- Butter, 2 tbsp.
- Pepper
- Salt
- Skin on, bone-in chicken thighs, 4

What to Do

- You need to warm your oven to 400.

- Put a skillet that can go into the oven on top of the stove on medium heat. Add in one tablespoon of butter. Sprinkle the chicken with pepper and salt.

- Lay the chicken in the skillet and brown on both sides. This will take about six minutes.

- Take thighs out of skillet and place to the side on a plate.
- Add the rest of the butter and add garlic until fragrant and translucent.
- Add lemon juice, heavy cream, and chicken stock. Mix well. Allow to boil and put the chicken back into the skillet.
- Cover and place into the oven for 30 minutes.

Stuffed Chicken Breast

This recipe makes 4 servings, and contains 389 calories; 30 grams fat; 25 grams protein; 3 grams net carbohydrates per serving

What You Need

- EVOO, 2 tbsp.
- Boneless, skin on chicken breasts, 4
- Chopped basil, 2 tbsp.
- Roasted, chopped bell pepper, .25 c
- Chopped Kalamata olives, .25 c
- Room temperature goat cheese, .5 c
- Chopped onion, .25 c
- Butter, 1 tbsp.

What to Do

- You need to warm your oven to 400.
- Place a skillet on top of the stove and melt butter on medium heat.
- Mix in the onion, cooking until translucent.
- Put the basil, bell pepper, olives, cheese, and onion into a blow. Mix well to combine. Place in the refrigerator for 30 minutes.
- Cut pockets into each of the chicken breasts, place the filling inside each breast. Secure with toothpicks.
- Using the same skillet, warm up the olive oil. Sear the chicken on each side.

- Place into the oven for 15 minutes. Chicken is done when it reaches an internal temperature of 165.
- Carefully remove toothpicks and enjoy.

Turkey Rissoles

This recipe makes 4 servings, and contains 440 calories; 34 grams fat; 27 grams protein; 3 grams net carbohydrates per serving

What You Need

- Olive oil, 2 tbsp.
- Ground almonds, 1 c
- Pepper
- Salt
- Minced garlic, 1 tsp.
- Chopped scallion, 1
- Ground turkey, 1 lb.

What to Do

- You need to warm your oven to 350.
- Place the pepper, salt, garlic, scallion, and turkey into a bowl. With your hands, mix everything together.
- Shape into eight patties and flatten.
- Place the almonds in a shallow bowl and put the patties into the almonds to coat. Press gently to make sure the almonds stick to the patties.
- Put a skillet onto the stove and warm the olive oil on medium heat. Place the patties into the skillet and cook for ten minutes on each side.
- Place aluminum foil onto a baking sheet. Lay the patties on a cooking sheet and slide into the oven. Bake for eight minutes. Turn oven and cook an additional eight minutes.

Stuffed Pork Chops

This recipe makes 4 servings, and contains 481 calories; 38 grams fat; 29 grams protein; 2 grams net carbohydrates per serving

What You Need

- Olive oil, 2 tbsp.
- Pepper
- Salt
- Butterflied pork chops, 4
- Chopped thyme, 1 tsp.
- Chopped almonds, .25 c
- Chopped walnuts, .5 c
- Goat cheese, 3 oz.

What to Do

- You need to warm your oven to 400.
- Put the thyme, almonds, walnuts, goat cheese into a bowl. Stir well to combine.
- Sprinkle pepper and salt on the pork chops on all sides. Spread the stuffing on one side of the pork chop. Fold the other side over and secure with toothpicks.
- Place a large skillet on top of the stove and warm the olive oil on medium heat. Sear the pork chops until browned on each side. This will take about ten minutes.
- Lay this in a baking dish and cook for 20 minutes.
- Carefully remove the toothpicks and enjoy.

Rosemary Garlic Rack of Lamb

This recipe makes 4 servings, and contains 354 calories; 30 grams fat; 21 grams protein; 0 gram net carbohydrates per serving

What You Need

- French-cut rack of lamb, 1 lb.
- Salt
- Minced garlic, 2 tsp.
- Chopped rosemary, 2 tbsp.
- EVOO, 4 tbsp.

What to Do

- Add the salt, garlic, rosemary, and olive oil into a bowl. Mix well to combine.
- Put the lamb into a zip-top bag and pour in the olive oil mixture. Rub the lamb with the mixture until coated. Press out as much air as you can get and make sure it is sealed.
- Refrigerate for at least two hours.
- To cook, take out of the refrigerator and let come to room temperature for 20 minutes.
- You need to warm your oven to 450.
- Put a skillet that can go into the oven on top of the stove and let it get hot. Sear the rack of lamb on each side. This will take about five minutes.
- Sit the rack upright in the skillet and interlace the bones. Place into the oven for about 20 minutes. This will get them to a medium rare consistency. The internal temp will be around 125.
- Allow to sit for ten minutes and cut into chops.
- Each person gets four chops.

Garlic Short Ribs

This recipe makes 4 servings, and contains 481 calories; 38 grams fat; 29 grams protein; 2 grams net carbohydrates per serving

What You Need

- Beef broth, 3 c
- Dry red wine, .5 c
- Minced garlic, 2 tsp.

- Olive oil, 1 tbsp.
- Pepper
- Salt
- Beef short ribs, 4 – 4 oz.

What to Do

- You need to warm your oven to 325.
- Sprinkle pepper and salt on the ribs on all sides.
- Put a large skillet that can go into the oven on top of the stove on medium heat and warm up the olive oil.
- Sear the ribs on every side and place on a plate.
- Using the same skillet, put the garlic in and cook until softened around three minutes.
- Add in the red wine and whisk to deglaze. Simmer until wine is reduced slightly.
- Add in ribs, juices on plate, and beef broth. And allow it to boil.
- Cover and put the skillet into the oven for two hours.
- Remove ribs onto a serving platter and drizzle with cooking liquid.

Bacon Wrapped Steaks

This recipe makes 4 servings, and contains 565 calories; 49 grams fat; 28 grams protein; 0 gram net carbohydrates per serving

What You Need

- Pepper
- Salt
- EVOO, 1 tbsp.
- Sliced bacon, 8
- Beef steaks, 4 – 4 oz.

What to Do

- You need to warm your oven to 450.
- Sprinkle each steak with pepper and salt generously.
- Wrap two slices of bacon around the edge of each steak. Secure with toothpicks.
- Place a large skillet on top of the stove and warm the olive oil.
- Sear the steaks on each side for four minutes. Place them on a cooking sheet.
- Bake them in the oven for six minutes for medium doneness.
- Take out of the oven and allow to rest for ten minutes.
- Carefully remove toothpicks and enjoy.

Italian Burgers

This recipe makes 4 servings, and contains 441 calories; 37 grams fat; 22 grams protein; 3 grams net carbohydrates per serving

What You Need

- Thinly sliced small onion
- Minced garlic, 1 tsp.
- Thickly sliced tomato
- Olive oil, 1 tbsp.
- Salt, .25 tsp.
- Chopped basil, 2 tbsp.
- Ground almonds, .25 c
- Ground beef, 1 lb.

What to Do

- Place the salt, garlic, basil, ground almonds, and ground beef into a bowl. Use your hand to combine all ingredients.
- Divide into four equal portions and form into patties. Flatten to about one-half inch thickness.
- Put a large cast iron skillet on top of the stove and warm the olive oil on medium heat.

- Place the burgers into the skillet and cook for six minutes on each side.
- Place onto paper towels to drain. Whisk away any grease that might form on the top of each burger with paper towels.
- Serve with onion and tomato.

Saffron Shrimp

This recipe makes 2 servings, and contains 333 calories; 13 grams fat; 45 grams protein; 9 grams net carbohydrates per serving

What You Need
- Lemon juice, 1 tbsp.
- Cayenne
- White pepper
- Chicken broth, .5 c
- Chopped tomato, 1
- Paprika
- Saffron
- Minced garlic, 2 cloves
- Cooked shrimp, 1 lb.
- Chopped fennel, .5
- Ghee, 2 tbsp.

What to Do
- Place a large skillet on top of the stove and melt the ghee on medium heat. Put the fennel into the skillet and cook until soft. Add in the paprika, saffron, garlic, and shrimp. Cook until shrimp is turning pink. If the skillet gets dry, add more ghee.
- Add in pepper, cayenne, lemon juice, broth, and tomato. Bring to simmer and let the liquid reduce for 20 minutes. Enjoy.

Pesto Chicken Casserole

This recipe makes 4 servings, and contains 512 calories; 110 grams fat; 42 grams protein; 7 grams net carbohydrates per serving

What You Need

- Pepper
- Salt
- Diced feta, 8 oz.
- Chopped garlic, 1 clove
- Chopped olives, .5 c
- Heavy whipping cream, 1.5 c
- Olive oil, 4 tbsp.
- Leafy greens, .75 c
- Chicken breasts, 1.5 lbs.
- Pesto, .33 c
- Butter, 4 tbsp.

What to Do

- You need to warm your oven to 450.
- Chop the chicken into cubes and sprinkle with pepper and salt.
- Place a skillet on top of the stove on medium heat and melt butter. Cook the chicken until browned do this in batches until all have been browned.
- Add the pesto and cream to a bowl and mix well to combine.
- Place the cooked chicken to the bottom of a casserole dish. Add in the olives, feta, and garlic. Drizzle the pesto over everything.
- Slide into the oven and cook for 25 minutes until the edges are browned and bubbly.

Meat Pie

This recipe makes 6 servings, and contains 133 calories; 47 grams fat; 38 grams protein; 7 grams net carbohydrates per serving

What You Need

- Chopped onion, .5
- Minced garlic, 1 clove
- Butter, 2 tbsp.
- Ground beef, 1.5 lb.
- Pepper
- Salt
- Water, .5 c
- Dried oregano, 1 tbsp.
- Tomato paste, 4 tbsp.
- For the Crust:
- Almond flour, .75 c
- Water, 4 tbsp.
- Sesame seeds, 4 tbsp.
- Egg, 1
- Coconut flour, 4 tbsp.
- Salt
- Ground psyllium husk powder, 1 tbsp.
- Baking powder, 1 tsp.
- For the Topping:
- Shredded cheese, 7 oz.
- Cottage cheese, 8 oz.

What to Do

- You need to warm your oven to 350.

- Place a skillet on top of the stove on medium and warm the butter. Mix in the garlic and onion, cooking until soft.

- Mix in the beef, cooking until completely browned. Add in the salt, basil, pepper, and oregano. Stir together.

- Pour in the water and tomato paste. Mix well. Lower heat and simmer 20 minutes. While cooking, make the crust.

- Add the dough ingredients to a food processor and mix until it forms a ball. You can do this by hand if you don't have a food processor.

- Take a springform pan and grease it generously. Place a piece of parchment paper into the bottom.

- Spread the dough onto the bottom and sides with your greased fingers.

- Place into the oven and bake for 15 minutes. Pour meat mixture into the crust.

- Mix the topping ingredients and spread on top of meat. Let the pie bake for 35 minutes until golden.

Soups

Cauliflower Soup

This recipe makes 8 servings, and contains 227 calories; 21 grams fat; 8 grams protein; 2 grams net carbohydrates per serving

What You Need

- Butter, .25 c
- Shredded cheddar, 1 c
- Pepper
- Salt
- Heavy cream, 1 c
- Nutmeg, .5 tsp.
- Chicken stock, 4 c
- Chopped cauliflower, 1 head
- Chopped onion, .5

What to Do

- Add the butter to a pot and melt.
- Cook the cauliflower and onion together for about ten minutes.
- Mix in the nutmeg and chicken stock and allow everything to come to a boil. Lower to a simmer and cook for 15 minutes.
- Mix in the heavy cream.
- Add the soup to a blender and puree until smooth. You may need to do this in more than one batch. Alternatively, you can use an immersion blender if you have on.
- Pour the soup back into the pot and season with some pepper and salt. Top with the cheese and serve.

Thai Chicken Soup

This recipe makes 4 servings, and contains 324 calories; 19 grams fat; 23 grams protein; 13 grams net carbohydrates per serving

What You Need

- Bunch cilantro
- Thai chili paste, 1 tsp.
- Lime juice, 2 tbsp.
- Cubed tomatoes, 2
- Sliced mushrooms, 1 c
- Thai fish sauce, 1 tbsp.
- Kaffir lime leaves, 6
- White parts from fresh lemongrass, 2 stalks – chopped and crushed
- Galangal, thumb-sized chunk
- Diced chicken thighs, 1 lb.
- Chicken broth, 14 oz.
- Coconut milk, 14 oz.

What to Do

- Add the lemongrass, sliced galangal, chili paste, broth, and coconut milk to a pot and heat up to medium-high. Allow this to come to a boil.
- Mix in the chicken and cook for another two minutes. Lower the heat.
- Mix in the tomatoes and mushrooms. Cook for another three to five minutes.
- Mix in the lime juice and fish sauce.
- Break up the lime leaves and stir them into the soup.
- Remove the galangal and lemongrass. Serve the soup topped with some fresh cilantro.

Bacon Cheeseburger Soup

This recipe makes 4 servings, and contains 758 calories; 57 grams fat; 48 grams protein; 11 grams net carbohydrates per serving

What You Need

- Pepper, .5 tsp.
- Salt, 2 tsp.
- Chili powder, 1 tsp.
- Onion powder, .5 tsp.
- Cream cheese, 3 oz.
- Dried parsley, 1 tsp.
- Heavy cream, .5 c
- Shredded cheddar, 1 c
- Beef broth, 4 c
- Butter, 3 tbsp.
- Garlic powder, .5 tsp.
- Bacon, 4 slices
- Ground beef, 1 lb.

What to Do

- Add the bacon to a large pot and cook until crispy. Lay it out on paper towels to drain.
- Add in the spices, beef, and butter. Let this cook until the beef has browned. Make sure you break it apart as it cooks.
- Add in the cheddar cheese, cream cheese, tomato paste, and broth. Stir until everything is melted and combined.
- Cook the soup, covered, on low for 25 minutes
- Sprinkle in some pepper and salt. Garnish the soup with the crumbled cooked bacon and some heavy cream.

Cheesy Broccoli Soup

This recipe makes 4 servings, and contains 185 calories; 14 grams fat; 10 grams protein; 4 grams net carbohydrates per serving

What You Need

- Pepper
- Salt
- Shredded cheddar, 1 c
- Broccoli, 3 c
- Heavy cream, .25 c
- Cream cheese, 1 tbsp.
- Chicken broth, 4 c
- Minced garlic, 2 cloves
- Diced small onion

What to Do

- Melt the butter in a pot and sauté the onions for three to four minutes. Mix in the garlic, cooking until fragrant.
- Mix in the broccoli and chicken broth.
- Allow the mixture to come to a boil and then reduce the heat so that it simmers for a few minutes.
- After the broccoli is soft, puree the soup with an immersion blender.
- Mix in the cream cheese and cream, stirring until well combined and melted.
- Take the pot off the heat and mix in the cheddar cheese. Enjoy.

Beef Stew

This recipe makes 4 servings, and contains 706 calories; 57 grams fat; 37 grams protein; 6 grams net carbohydrates per serving

What You Need

- Pepper
- Salt
- Almond flour, .25 c
- Thyme, 1 tbsp.
- Worcestershire sauce, 1 tbsp.
- Beef broth, 1 c
- Diced tomatoes, 3
- Minced garlic, 2 cloves
- Hot sauce, 2 tsp.
- Chopped onion, .5
- 1-inch cube beef stew meat, 2 lbs.

What to Do

- Turn your slow cooker to the high settings.
- Mix the almond flour with some pepper and salt. Coat the stew meat in the flour. Lay the meat in your slow cooker.
- Pour in the remaining ingredients.
- Set to cook for 30 minutes on high, then, switch to low and cook for six hours.
- Adjust the flavorings as you see fit.

Chicken Soup

This recipe makes 8 servings, and contains 285 calories; 40 grams fat; 33 grams protein; 4 grams net carbohydrates per serving

What You Need

- Butter, .5 c

- Celery stalks, 2
- Dried parsley, 2 tsp.
- Sliced mushrooms, 6 oz.
- Minced garlic, 2 cloves
- Dried onion, 2 tbsp.
- Salt, 1 tsp.
- Chicken broth, 8 c
- Sliced cabbage, 2 c
- Pepper, .25 tsp.
- Shredded, cooked chicken, 2 c
- Medium Carrot

What to Do

- Place a large stock pot to the stove on medium and melt butter. Slice the celery and carrots.
- Put the dried onion, mushrooms, celery, and garlic into the pot and cook for four minutes.
- Add in salt, parsley, pepper, chicken, broth, and carrot. Allow this to boil for 12 minutes or until cabbage is tender.

Easy Chicken Chili

This recipe makes 4 servings, and contains 421 calories; 21 grams fat; 45 grams protein; 6 grams net carbohydrates per serving

What You Need

- Pepper
- Salt
- Cream cheese, 4 oz.
- Chili powder, 1 tbsp.

- Serrano pepper, 1
- Garlic powder, .5 tbsp.
- Cumin, 1 tbsp.
- Tomato puree, 2 oz.
- Diced tomatoes, 8 oz.
- Chicken broth, 2 c
- Onion, .5
- Butter, 1 tbsp.
- Boneless, skinless, chicken breasts, 4

What to Do

- Take the chicken breasts and cut them into cubes.
- Place a large pan on medium heat. Pour water into a pan and allow to boil. Add chicken into the water and boil until cooked through about ten minutes. Remove chicken from pan and set to the side. Pour water out of the pan and place back onto heat.
- Add butter to melt. Add onion and cook until softened. Put chicken back into the pot along with the chili powder, broth, tomato puttee, garlic, Serrano pepper, cumin, and tomatoes. Let everything boil. Turn to a simmer for ten minutes.
- While chili is simmering, cut the cream cheese into chunks and place in the pan. Stirring until melted.
- Ladle into bowls and enjoy.

Turkey and Leek Soup

This recipe makes 4 servings, and contains 305 calories; 11 grams fat; 15 grams protein; 3 grams net carbohydrates per serving

What You Need

- Shredded turkey, 3 c
- Chopped zoodles, 3 c
- Chopped parsley, .25 c

- Pepper
- Salt
- Chicken broth, 6 c
- Butter, 1 tbsp.
- Chopped leeks, 2
- Chopped celery, 3

What to Do

- Place a large stock pot on medium and melt butter. Add in celery and leeks, cooking until softened for about five minutes.
- Add in chicken broth, pepper, salt, turkey meat, and parsley into the pot. Once this comes to a boil, turn to a simmer for 20 minutes.
- Add in the zoodles and cook an additional five minutes.
- Ladle into bowls and enjoy.

Turkey Chili

This recipe makes 5 servings, and contains 295 calories; 15 grams fat; 25 grams protein; 4 grams net carbohydrates per serving

What You Need

- Chili powder, 2 tbsp.
- Pepper
- Salt
- Cumin, 1 tbsp.
- Turmeric, 1 tbsp.
- Grated ginger, 2 tbsp.
- Coconut oil, 2 tbsp.
- Coriander, 1 tbsp.
- Sliced onions, 2

- Minced garlic, 2 cloves
- Coconut cream, 2 tbsp.
- Diced tomatoes, 20 oz.
- Kale, 3 oz.
- Cooked and shredded turkey breasts, 18 oz.

What to Do

- Place a large pot on medium and melt coconut oil. Add the onion, cooking until soft. Mix in ginger and garlic and cook until fragrant about one minute.
- Put the chili powder, cumin, salt, coriander, turmeric, pepper, and tomatoes into the pot and stir well to combine. Add in the coconut cream. Bring to boil and cook ten minutes.
- Add in the kale and turkey breasts. Allow this to boil and then simmer for another 15 minutes.

Turkey Stew

This recipe makes 6 servings, and contains 193 calories; 11 grams fat; 27 grams protein; 2 grams net carbohydrates per serving

What You Need

- Chopped cilantro, 1 tbsp.
- Sour cream, .25 c
- Cumin, 2 tsp.
- Coriander, 1 tsp.
- Salsa verde, .5 c
- Garlic powder, .5 tsp.
- Chopped canned chipotle peppers, 1 tbsp.
- Pepper
- Salt

- Chicken broth, 6 c
- Green beans, 2 c
- Shredded, cooked turkey meat, 4 c

What to Do

- Add the broth to a pot.
- Add the green beans, cooking for ten minutes.
- Mix in the pepper, cumin, chipotles, salsa verde, salt, coriander, garlic powder, and turkey. Stir well and cook another ten minutes.
- Add in sour cream and give everything a good stir. Take off heat and divide into bowls. Sprinkle with cilantro and serve.

Coconut Chicken Soup

This recipe makes 4 servings, and contains 387 calories; 23 grams fat; 31 grams protein; 5 grams net carbohydrates per serving

What You Need

- Chopped celery, .25 c
- Coconut cream, .5 c
- Pepper
- Salt
- Chicken broth, 4 c
- Diced chicken breasts, 2
- Cream cheese, 4 oz.
- Butter, 3 tbsp.

What to Do

- Melt the butter in a large pot. Add in celery, cooking until soft. Mix in the pepper, salt, cream cheese, and coconut cream. Stir until cream cheese is melted and everything is well incorporated.

- Stir in chicken and simmer for 15 minutes.
- Ladle into bowls and serve.

Mexican Turkey Soup

This recipe makes 4 servings, and contains 387 calories; 24 grams fat; 38 grams protein; 6 grams net carbohydrates per serving

What You Need

- Chunked cheddar, 8 oz.
- Chunky salsa, 15 oz.
- Chicken broth, 15 oz.
- Cubed turkey thighs, 1.5 lbs.

What to Do

- Put everything in a slow cooker and mix.
- Cover, turn to high and cook for four hours. You can also cook this on low for eight hours.
- Gently remove the lid, stir well to incorporate the cheese.
- Ladle into bowls and serve.

Sun-Dried Tomato and Chicken Stew

This recipe makes 4 servings, and contains 224 calories; 11 grams fat; 23 grams protein; 6 grams net carbohydrates per serving

What You Need

- Pepper
- Salt
- Heavy cream, .5 c
- Thyme, .25 tsp.

- Oregano, .5 tsp.
- Spinach, 1 c
- Chopped sun-dried tomatoes, 2 oz.
- Rosemary, .5 tsp.
- Minced garlic, 3 cloves
- Cubed chicken thighs, 28 oz.
- Chopped shallot, 1
- Chicken broth, 2 c
- Chopped celery, 2
- Chopped carrots, 2
- Xanthan gum, pinch

What to Do

- Heat up a large pot and add in the pepper, oregano, garlic, celery, onion, thyme, salt, rosemary, carrots, tomatoes, broth, and chicken. Stir well to combine.
- Let this come to a boil and then turn to a simmer for 45 minutes.
- Do a taste test and adjust pepper and salt if needed. Add in the spinach, xanthan gum, and cream. Cook an additional ten minutes.
- Ladle into bowls and serve.

Cream of Tomato and Thyme Soup

This recipe makes 6 servings, and contains 310 calories; 27 grams fat; 11 grams protein; 3 grams net carbohydrates per serving

What You Need

- Heavy cream, 1 c
- Pepper
- Salt
- Water, 1.5 c

- Thyme leaves, 1 tsp.
- Canned tomatoes, 2 – 28 oz.
- Diced cashews, .5 c
- Diced onion, 2 large
- Ghee, 2 tbsp.

What to Do

- Melt the ghee in a large pot. Add in the onion and cook until soft.
- Add in pepper, salt, cashews, water, thyme, and tomatoes. Stir to combine. Bring to boil. Cover with a lid and simmer it for ten minutes.
- Take the lid off. Use an immersion blender to process until smooth. Taste and adjust if necessary. Add in the heavy cream, stir well to combine.
- Ladle into bowls and serve.

Gazpacho

This recipe makes 6 servings, and contains 528 calories; 46 grams fat; 8 grams protein; 8 grams net carbohydrates per serving

What You Need

- Salt
- Apple cider vinegar, 2 tbsp.
- Chopped onion, 1 small
- Goat cheese, 7 oz.
- Chopped tomatoes, 4
- Roasted green bell peppers, 2
- Lemon juice, 2 tbsp.
- Olive oil, 1 c
- Chopped cucumber, 1
- Chopped green onion, 2

- Garlic, 2 cloves
- Avocados, 2
- Roasted red bell peppers, 2

What to Do

- Place the salt, vinegar, olive oil, lemon juice, garlic, onion, avocado, tomatoes, and peppers into a blender or food processor. Process until either completely smooth or slightly chunky. Whichever you would prefer.
- Taste and adjust seasonings as needed.
- Place into an airtight container. Add in the green onions and cucumbers. Refrigerate for no less than two hours.
- When ready to eat, ladle into bowls.
- Top with a drizzle of olive oil and goat cheese.

Coconut and Shrimp Curry Soup

This recipe makes 4 servings, and contains 375 calories; 35 grams fat; 9 grams protein; 2 grams net carbohydrates per serving

What You Need

- Halved green beans, 1 bunch
- Chili pepper
- Salt
- Coconut milk, 6 oz.
- Red curry paste, 2 tbsp.
- Ginger garlic pureed, 2 tsp.
- Peeled and deveined jumbo shrimp, 1 lb.
- Ghee, 2 tbsp.

What to Do

- Place a skillet on medium and melt ghee. Add in the shrimp and sprinkle with pepper and salt. Cool until turning slightly pink. Take out of the skillet and put on a plate. Set to the side.

- Add the red curry paste and ginger garlic puree to the same skillet and cook until fragrant.

- Add in the green beans, chili pepper, salt, coconut milk, and place the shrimp back into the skillet. Stir well to combine. Cook an additional four minutes. Lower heat and simmer another three minutes, stir occasionally.

- Adjust any of the seasonings that you need to.

- Ladle into bowls and serve with some cauli-rice if desired.

Green Minestrone Soup

This recipe makes 4 servings, and contains 227 calories; 20 grams fat; 8 grams protein; 2 grams net carbohydrates per serving

What You Need

- Pepper
- Salt
- Baby spinach, 1 c
- Vegetable broth, 5 c
- Chopped celery, 2
- Chopped broccoli, 2 heads
- Onion garlic puree, 2 tbsp.
- Ghee, 2 tbsp.

What to Do

- Place a saucepan on medium and melt ghee. Add in the onion-garlic puree and cook until warmed.

- Mix in the celery and broccoli and cook until tender.

- Pour in broth and stir everything together. Let this come up to a boil. Lower the heat and cook while covered for five minutes.

- Add spinach in batches until wilted. Add pepper and salt to taste and cook four more minutes. Taste and adjust seasoning if needed.
- Ladle into bowls and sprinkle with Gruyere cheese if desired. Can be eaten with a low carb bread.

Shrimp Stew

This recipe makes 6 servings, and contains 324 calories; 21 grams fat; 23 grams protein; 5 grams net carbohydrates per serving

What You Need
- Pepper
- Salt
- Chopped Dill
- Chopped cilantro, .25 c
- Chopped onions, .25 c
- Sriracha sauce, 2 tbsp.
- Diced tomatoes, 14 oz.
- Minced garlic, 1 clove
- Olive oil, .25 c
- Peeled, deveined shrimp, 1.5 lb.
- Diced roasted peppers, .25 c
- Lime juice, 2 tbsp.
- Coconut milk, 1 c

What to Do
- Place a pot on medium and warm olive oil. Mix in the onion, cooking until translucent.
- Mix in garlic, cooking until fragrant.
- Add in cilantro, shrimp, and tomatoes. Cook until shrimp turns pink.

- Stir in coconut milk and Sriracha and cook a few more minutes. Don't boil just warm through. Add in lime juice and sprinkle with pepper and salt. Taste and adjust any seasonings as needed.
- Ladle into bowls, sprinkle with fresh dill and serve.

Sausage Beer Soup

This recipe makes 8 servings, and contains 244 calories; 17 grams fat; 5 grams protein; 4 grams net carbohydrates per serving

What You Need
- Chopped cilantro
- Pepper
- Salt
- Cheddar cheese, 1 c
- Diced onion, 1
- Chopped celery, 1 c
- Beef broth, 2 c
- Beer, 6 oz.
- Red pepper flakes, 1 tsp.
- Cream cheese, 8 oz.
- Minced garlic, 4 cloves
- Chopped carrots, 1 c
- Sliced beef sausages, 10 oz.
- Heavy cream, 1 c

What to Do
- Turn your slow cooker to low.

- Add the pepper, salt, red pepper flakes, salt, celery, onion, carrots, sausage, beer, and broth into the slow cooker. Stir well to combine. Add in just enough water to cover the ingredients by two inches.

- Put the lid on the cooker and set the timer for six hours.

- Carefully remove the lid and add in the cream cheese, cheddar, and heavy cream. Stir well. Place the lid back on and cook an additional two hours.

- When done, stir well to combine. Taste and adjust seasonings if needed.

- Ladle into bowls, sprinkle with cilantro and serve.

Wild Mushroom and Thyme Soup

This recipe makes 4 servings, and contains 281 calories; 25 grams fat; 6 grams protein; 6 grams net carbohydrates per serving

What You Need

- Pepper
- Salt
- Chicken broth, 4 c
- Minced garlic, 2 cloves
- Thyme leaves, 2 tsp.
- Chopped wild mushrooms, 12 oz.
- Crème Fraiche, 5 oz.
- Butter, .25 c

What to Do

- Melt the ghee in a large pot. Add in the garlic and cook until fragrant. Put the mushrooms into the pot and sprinkle with pepper and salt. Cook for ten minutes. Add in broth and allow to boil.

- Lower heat and simmer ten minutes. Use an immersion blender and process until smooth. You can also use a blender if you don't have an immersion blender.

- Put the crème Fraiche in and stir well.

- Ladle into bowls and garnish with thyme.

Reuben Soup

This recipe makes 7 servings, and contains 450 calories; 37 grams fat; 23 grams protein; 8 grams net carbohydrates per serving

What You Need

- Pepper
- Salt
- Swiss cheese, 1.5 c
- Butter, 3 tbsp.
- Chopped corned beef, 1 lb.
- Sauerkraut, 1 c
- Heavy cream, 2 c
- Minced garlic, 2 cloves
- Diced celery, 2
- Caraway seeds, 1 tsp.
- Diced onion, 1

What to Do

- Place a large pot on medium and melt butter. Mix in the onion and celery, cooking until tender. Mix in the garlic and cook until fragrant.
- Add in broth, pepper, caraway seeds, salt, and sauerkraut. Stir well. Allow to boil. Lower heat and put corned beef into the pot.
- Simmer for 15 minutes. Taste and adjust seasonings if needed.
- Add in cheese and heavy cream and cook one more minute.

Salads

Taco Salad

This recipe makes 4 servings, and contains 516 calories; 37 grams fat; 35 grams protein; 5 grams net carbohydrates per serving

What You Need

- Water, .5 c
- Cumin, 1.5 tsp.
- Paprika, .5 tsp.
- Oregano, .25 tsp.
- Garlic powder, .25 tsp.
- Ground beef, 1 lb.
- Sliced onion, 2 tbsp.
- Salt, 1 tsp.
- Sour cream, .5 c
- Olive oil, 1 tbsp.
- Juice of lime, .5
- Avocado
- Chopped tomato
- Chopped lettuce, 2 c
- Grated cheese, .5 c

What to Do

- Add the beef to a skillet and brown. This will take about eight to ten minutes.
- Mix in the cumin, paprika, oregano, garlic powder, and ½ cup of water. Allow this to simmer for three minutes, or until the water has evaporated.
- Toss together the onion, avocado, and lettuce.
- Mix in the salt, lime juice, and oil.

- Top with the beef, cheese, tomatoes, and sour cream.

Crab Salad Avocado

This recipe makes 2 servings, and contains 389 calories; 31 grams fat; 19 grams protein; 5 grams net carbohydrates per serving

What You Need

- Pepper
- Salt
- Chopped cilantro, 1 tsp.
- Chopped scallion, .5
- Chopped English cucumber, .25 c
- Chopped red bell pepper, .25 c
- Cream cheese, .5 c
- Crab meat, 4.5 oz.
- Lemon juice, .5 tsp.
- Halved avocado

What to Do

- Brush the avocado with the lemon so that it doesn't become brown. Lay them on a plate cut side up.
- Mix together the pepper, salt, cilantro, scallion, cucumber, red pepper, crab meat, and cream cheese.
- Divide the crabmeat mixture between the two avocado halves and serve.

Tuna Salad

This recipe makes 2 servings, and contains 465 calories; 18 grams fat; 68 grams protein; 6 grams net carbohydrates per serving

What You Need

- Salt, 1 tsp.
- Mayonnaise, 2 tbsp.
- EVOO, 1 tbsp.
- Lemon juice, 2 tbsp.
- Chopped cilantro, .5 bunch
- Sliced small onion
- Dijon, 2 tsp.
- Sliced cucumber, .5
- Chopped boiled eggs, 2
- Drained tuna in oil, 2 15-oz. can

What to Do

- Mix together the salt, olive oil, lemon juice, Dijon, and mayonnaise.
- Toss everything together. Top with the dressing and toss everything together. Enjoy.

BLT Salad

This recipe makes 4 servings, and contains 228 calories; 18 grams fat; 1 gram protein; 2 grams net carbohydrates per serving

What You Need

- Sliced cooked chicken breast
- Toasted sesame seeds, 1 tsp.
- Chopped hardboiled egg, 2
- Chopped cooked bacon, 6 slices
- Chopped tomato
- Sunflower seeds, 1 tbsp.
- Shredded lettuce, 4 c

- Pepper
- Red wine vinegar, 2 tbsp.
- Bacon fat, 2 tbsp.

What to Do

- Whisk the vinegar and bacon fat together until emulsified. Add in the pepper.
- Toss the tomato and lettuce into the dressing.
- Divide this between four plates and top each with chicken, sesame seeds, sunflower seeds, egg, and bacon.

Salmon Salad

This recipe makes 2 servings, and contains 492 calories; 39 grams fat; 25 grams protein; 7 grams net carbohydrates per serving

What You Need

- Pepper, .5 tsp.
- Salt, .25 tsp.
- Olive oil, 2 tbsp.
- Chopped walnuts, .25 c
- Diced avocado
- Smoked salmon, 7 oz.
- Lemon juice, 2 tbsp.
- Mixed leafy greens, 6 oz.

What to Do

- Add the pepper, salt, avocado, and leafy greens to a bowl and toss everything together.
- Add in the lemon juice and olive oil and mix everything together.
- Divide into two serving bowls and top with the walnuts and salmon.

Feta Salad

This recipe makes 2 servings, and contains 619 calories; 59 grams fat; 13 grams protein; 8 grams net carbohydrates per serving

What You Need

- Salt, .5 tsp.
- EVOO, .25 c
- Pepper, .25 tsp.
- Dijon, 1 tsp.
- Balsamic vinegar, 2 tbsp.
- Bacon, 2 slices
- Feta, 3 oz.
- Walnut pieces, .5 c
- Mixed salad greens, 2 c

What to Do

- Cook the bacon until crispy.
- Mix the walnuts, cheese, and greens together. Crumble up the bacon and toss into the greens.
- Beat together the pepper, salt, mustard, and balsamic vinegar. Whisk the dressing as you pour in the olive oil until well blended.
- Dress the salad and toss everything together. Serve.

Turkey and Avocado Salad

This recipe makes 4 servings, and contains 559 calories; 30 grams fat; 60 grams protein; 5 grams net carbohydrates per serving

What You Need

- Pepper
- Salt
- Sliced cherry tomatoes, 12
- Mustard, 1 tbsp.
- Olive oil, 2 tbsp.
- Spinach, 7 c
- Cubed avocado, 1 c
- Crumbled feta, 1 c
- Chopped cooked turkey bacon, 3 slices
- Diced grilled turkey breasts, 2 lb.

What to Do

- Mix together the oil, mustard, and a tablespoon of water. Stir in some pepper and salt. Set to the side.
- Toss the spinach in half of the dressing.
- Add in the tomatoes, cheese, avocado, turkey, and bacon.
- Add in the rest of the dressing and sprinkle in some pepper and salt. Enjoy.

Caesar Salad

This recipe makes 2 servings, and contains 734 calories; 58 grams fat; 41 grams protein; 6 grams net carbohydrates per serving

What You Need

- Homemade Caesar dressing, 2 tbsp.
- Parmesan, 1 tbsp.
- Romaine lettuce, 4 c
- Bacon, 1 c

- Sliced avocado
- Grilled chicken breast, 10 oz.

For the Dressing
- Lemon juice, 2 tbsp.
- Garlic clove
- Pepper
- Salt
- Mayonnaise, .5 c
- Dijon, 1.5 tsp.

What to Do
- To make the salad dressing, add everything to a blender and combine until smooth.
- To make the salad, cook the chopped bacon and heat until crispy.
- Mix together the cooked bacon, chicken, and sliced avocado.
- Drizzle the salad with the Caesar dressing. Top with some Parmesan and enjoy.

Brussels Sprouts Salad

This recipe makes 1 serving, and contains 282 calories; 28 grams fat; 3 grams protein; 5 grams net carbohydrates per serving

What You Need
- Pepper
- Lemon juice, 1 tbsp.
- EVOO, 2 tbsp.
- Chopped Brussels, 1 c

What to Do

- Place the lemon juice, olive oil, and Brussels into a bowl. Toss to coat. Sprinkle on some pepper, taste and adjust seasoning if needed.

Avocado Salad

This recipe makes 4 servings, and contains 285 calories; 123 grams fat; 27 grams protein; 6 grams net carbohydrates per serving

What You Need

- Goat cheese, 8 oz.
- Sliced bacon, 8 oz.
- Avocados, 2
- Arugula, .5 c
- Walnuts, 4 oz.
- For Dressing:
- Juice of .5 lemon
- Heavy whipping cream, 2 tbsp.
- Mayonnaise, .5 c
- Olive oil, .5 c

What to Do

- You need to warm your oven to 400. Use parchment paper to line a baking dish.
- Slice the goat cheese into slices that are one half inches thick and lay in the baking dish.
- Place into the oven and bake until golden.
- Place a skillet on top of the stove and cook the bacon until crispy.
- Slice the avocados in half and carefully remove the pit. Scoop out and slice.
- Divide the arugula evenly between four plates. Add the sliced avocado on top. Place the bacon and goat cheese on top. Sprinkle with walnuts.
- Add the dressing ingredients to a blender and mix until smooth. Add in some pepper and salt. Serve with a drizzle of dressing.

Tuna Salad

This recipe makes 2 servings, and contains 387 calories; 91 grams fat; 33 grams protein; 6 grams net carbohydrates per serving

What You Need

- Pepper
- Salt
- Romaine lettuce, .5 lb.
- Dijon mustard, 1 tsp.
- Cherry tomatoes, 4 oz.
- Eggs, 4
- Juice and zest from .5 lemon
- Scallions, 2
- Olive oil, 2 tbsp.
- Mayonnaise, .75 c
- Celery stalks, 4 oz.
- Tuna, 5 oz.

What to Do

- Finely chop the celery and scallions. Combine the lemon zest, lemon juice, mayonnaise, mustard, celery, scallions, and tuna. Add pepper and salt. Set to the side.
- Put the eggs into a pot and cover with water. Let the eggs boil for six minutes for soft or medium eggs or ten minutes for hardboiled.
- Place the eggs into ice water and peel once cooled. Cut them in half.
- Put the lettuce onto tow bowls and top with the tuna mixture and eggs. Top with tomatoes and drizzle with some olive oil. Sprinkle with pepper and salt.

Turkey Salad

This recipe makes 4 servings, and contains 451 calories; 33 grams fat; 28 grams protein; 6 grams net carbohydrates per serving

What You Need

For Salad

- Halved pecans, .5 c
- Raspberries, .5 pint
- Pepper
- Salt
- Crumbled goat cheese, 4 oz.
- Turkey breasts, 2
- Baby spinach, 10 oz.

For Vinaigrette

- Pepper
- Salt
- Dijon mustard, 1 tbsp.
- Raspberries .75 c
- Water, .25 c
- Olive oil, .25 c
- Vinegar, .25 c
- Chopped onion, 1
- Swerve, 1 tbsp.

What to Do

- Place the salt, oil, onion, water, mustard, pepper, raspberries, vinegar, and swerve into a blender. Process until well blended. Press the mixture through a mesh sieve to get rid of the seeds. Set to the side.

- Season the turkey breast with pepper and salt. Put a skillet on medium heat and place turkey into the skillet.

- Cook eight minutes, turn over and cook another eight minutes.

- Take the goat cheese, pecan halves, raspberries, and spinach and divide it evenly between four bowls. Slice the turkey breasts and add them to the top of the salad. Drizzle on the vinaigrette and enjoy.

Steak Salad

This recipe makes 4 servings, and contains 325 calories; 19 grams fat; 28 grams protein; 4 grams net carbohydrates per serving

What You Need

For the Dressing

- Red wine vinegar, 1 tbsp.
- Pepper
- Salt
- Erythritol, 1 tsp.
- Olive oil, 3 tbsp. + extra to drizzle
- Dijon mustard, 2 tsp.

For Salad

- Pepper
- Salt
- Mixed salad greens, 2 c
- Water, .5 c
- Chopped kohlrabi, 2

- Chopped green beans, 1 c
- Sliced tomatoes, 3
- Sliced green onions, 3
- Rump steak, .5 lb., fat trimmed

What to Do

- You need to warm your oven to 400. Put the kohlrabi on a baking sheet and coat with the oil. Put into the oven for 25 minutes.
- Once cooked, allow it to cook.
- Mix the olive oil, vinegar, pepper, salt, erythritol, and Dijon mustard together. Whisk to combine. Set to the side.
- Preheat a cast iron skillet. Rub the steaks with pepper and salt. Put steaks into the skillet and sear on each side. Continue to cook until steaks are to your desired doneness. Let the steak rest for five minutes before slicing.
- In salad bowls, add the sliced steak, greens, kohlrabi, green beans, tomatoes, and green onions. Drizzle with dressing and toss to combine.
- Serve warm with some low carb bread if desired.

Tuna Caprese Salad

This recipe makes 4 servings, and contains 360 calories; 31 grams fat; 21 grams protein; 1 gram net carbohydrates per serving

What You Need

- Juice of one lemon
- EVOO, 2 tbsp.
- Pitted and sliced black olives, .5 c
- Basil, 6 leaves
- Sliced mozzarella, 8 oz.
- Sliced tomatoes, 2
- Chunked tuna in water, 2 – 10 oz. cans, drained

What to Do

- Put the drained tuna into the middle of a serving platter. Place the tomato slices and cheese around tuna. Alternate a slice of cheese, tomato, and basil leaf until all the way around the platter.

- Sprinkle the black olives on top and drizzle with lemon juice and olive oil.

Asian Beef Salad

This recipe makes 2 servings, and contains 385 calories; 98 grams fat; 34 grams protein; 7 grams net carbohydrates per serving

What You Need

For Steaks

- Grated ginger, 1 tbsp.
- Olive oil, 1 tbsp.
- Chili flakes, 1 tsp.
- Fish sauce, 1 tbsp.
- Ribeye steak, .66 lb.

For Salad

- Scallions, 2
- Cherry tomatoes, 3 oz.
- Cucumber, 2
- Lettuce, 1 head
- Red onion, .5
- Cilantro
- Sesame seeds, 1 tbsp.
- For Mayo:

- Pepper
- Salt
- Lime juice, .5 tbsp.
- Olive oil, .5 c
- Sesame oil, 1 tbsp.
- Egg yolk
- Dijon mustard, 1 tsp.

What to Do

- Make the mayo: Add the egg yolk and mustard into a bowl and whisk together. While whisking, slowly add in olive oil. You can do this by hand or using an immersion blender. After the mayo is emulsified, add in spices, sesame oil, and lime juice. Place this to the side.
- For the steak: Mix the fish sauce, ginger, chili flakes, and olive oil together. Add to a large zip-top bag. Place ribeye into the mixture and marinate it for 15 minutes.
- While steak is marinating, chop all vegetables for the salad except scallions. Divide these evenly between two plates
- Place a skillet on medium heat, put the sesame seeds into the skillet and let them roast for a few minutes. Put these to the side.
- Remove ribeye from the bag and pat dry. Place in the same skillet and sear on all sides. Continue to cook until it is done to your liking. This cut of meat is best at medium.
- Place the scallions to the skillet and cook them for a few minutes.
- Slice the steak thinly. Add the scallions and beef to the tops of the vegetables. Sprinkle with sesame seeds. Serve with the mayo as dressing.

Bacon and Blue Cheese Salad

This recipe makes 4 servings, and contains 205 calories; 20 grams fat; 4 grams protein; 2 grams net carbohydrates per serving

What You Need

- Pepper
- Salt

- EVOO, 3 tbsp.
- White wine vinegar, 1 tbsp.
- Crumbled blue cheese, 1.5 c
- Sliced bacon, 8
- Mixed salad greens, 2 – 8 oz. bags

What to Do

- Place the salad greens into a salad bowl. Set to the side.
- Cook the bacon in a skillet on medium until crisp. Place on paper towels to drain. Let cool until able to crumble with hands. Once crumbled, sprinkle on top of greens. Add in half the blue cheese, and toss to combine. Set to the side.
- In a small bowl, whisk the pepper, salt, olive, and vinegar until combined. Drizzle about half over salad, toss again, and add remaining cheese.
- Divide into four plates and serve with more dressing if desired.

Prawn Salad

This recipe makes 4 servings, and contains 215 calories; 20 grams fat; 8 grams protein; 2 grams net carbohydrates per serving

What You Need

For Dressing

- Lemon juice, 2 tbsp.
- Garlic mayonnaise, .5 c
- Dijon mustard, 1 tsp.

For Salad

- Chili Pepper
- Salt

- Peeled and deveined tiger prawns, 1 lb.
- Olive oil, 3 tbsp.
- Baby arugula, 4 c

What to Do

- Whisk the mustard, lemon juice, and mayonnaise together. Place in the refrigerator until ready to use.
- Place a skillet on medium and warm two tablespoons olive oil. Lay the prawns in a bowl and top with chili pepper and salt. Toss to coat. Place in the olive oil and cook until pink. Take out of skillet and place on a plate to be used later.
- Put the arugula in a serving bowl and pour about half the dressing on top. Toss and add the rest of the dressing if desired.
- Place the salad on four plates, top with prawns, and serve.

Garlicky Chicken Salad

This recipe makes 4 servings, and contains 286 calories; 23 grams fat; 14 grams protein; 4 grams net carbohydrates per serving

What You Need

- Crumbled blue cheese, 1 c
- Red wine vinegar, 1 tbsp.
- Garlic powder, 2 tbsp.
- Mixed salad greens, 1.5 c
- Olive oil, 1 tsp.
- Pepper
- Salt
- Skinless, boneless, chicken breasts, 2

What to Do

- Place the chicken breasts between two pieces of saran wrap. Beat the breasts with a meat mallet or rolling pin. Season with garlic powder, pepper, and salt.

- Place a cast iron skillet on high and warm oil. Fry the chicken four minutes on both sides until golden. It needs to reach 165. Place cooked chicken on a cutting board and let cool before slicing.

- Toss greens with red wine vinegar and divide evenly between four plates. Divide the chicken between the four salads and sprinkle with blue cheese. Serve.

Strawberry Spinach Salad

This recipe makes 2 servings, and contains 445 calories; 34 grams fat; 33 grams protein; 5 grams net carbohydrates per serving

What You Need

- Pepper
- Salt
- Raspberry vinaigrette, 4 tbsp.
- Grated goat cheese, 1.5 c
- Flaked almonds, .5 c
- Sliced strawberries, 4
- Spinach, 4 c

What to Do

- You need to warm your oven to 400. Place two pieces of parchment paper and place it on a baking sheet. Place the goat cheese into two circles. Put into the oven for ten minutes.

- Find two bowls that are the same size and put them upside down. Carefully place the parchment on top of the bowls to form the cheese into bowls. Let sit for 15 minutes.

- Once bowls have hardened, divide the spinach between the bowls. Drizzle the top with vinaigrette. Sprinkle on strawberries and almonds.

- Add in the green beans, chili pepper, salt, coconut milk, and place the shrimp back into the skillet. Stir well to combine. Cook an additional four minutes. Lower heat and simmer another three minutes, occasionally stirring.

- Adjust any seasonings that you need.

- Ladle into bowls and serve with some cauli-rice if desired.

Warm Artichoke Salad

This recipe makes 4 servings, and contains 170 calories; 13 grams fat; 1 gram protein; 5 grams net carbohydrates per serving

What You Need

- Caper brine, .25 tsp.
- Capers, 1 tbsp.
- Pepper, .25 tsp.
- Salt, .5 tsp.
- Lemon zest, .25 tsp.
- Chopped dill, 1 tbsp.
- Balsamic vinegar, 2 tsp.
- Olive oil, .25 c
- Sliced olives, .25 c
- Halved cherry peppers, .25 c
- Water, 6 c
- Baby artichokes, 6

What to Do

- Pour the water into a pot and add salt. Place on medium.
- Trim the artichokes and cut them in half and add to the pot. Allow to boil.
- Lower the heat and simmer 20 minutes until tender.
- Place the remaining ingredients into a bowl except for the olives. Stir well to combine.
- Drain the artichokes and put them onto a serving plate.
- Pour the vinaigrette over the artichokes and toss.
- Top with sliced olives.

Spinach Bacon Salad

This recipe makes 4 servings, and contains 350 calories; 33 grams fat; 7 grams protein; 3 grams net carbohydrates per serving

What You Need

For Salad

- Chopped hard-boiled eggs, 2
- Chopped lettuce, 2 small
- Spinach, 2 c
- Cooked, crumbled bacon, 4 slices
- Sliced green onion, 1
- Sliced avocado, 1
- Chopped avocado, 1

For Vinaigrette

- Dijon mustard, 1 tsp.
- Apple cider vinegar, 1 tbsp.
- Olive oil, 3 tbsp.

What to Do

- Into a large bowl, place green onion, chopped avocado, eggs, lettuce, and spinach. Toss to combine.
- Whisk the vinaigrette ingredients together.
- Pour the dressing on the salad and toss again to coat.
- Divide out into four plates and top with crumbled bacon and sliced avocados.

Crab Meat Salad

This recipe makes 4 servings, and contains 182 calories; 15 grams fat; 12 grams protein; 2 grams net carbohydrates per serving

What You Need

For Salad

- Chopped dill, 1 tbsp.
- Crab meat, 2 c
- Sliced black olives, .5 c
- Diced celery, .33 c
- Cauliflower, 5 c

For Dressing

- Salt
- Swerve, 2 tsp.
- Lemon juice, 2 tbsp.
- Pepper
- Celery seeds, .25 tsp.
- Apple cider vinegar, 1 tsp.
- Mayonnaise, .5 c

What to Do

- Put the dill, shrimp, celery, and cauliflower into a large bowl.
- In a small bowl, add the lemon juice, sweetener, celery seeds, vinegar, and mayonnaise. Whisk to combine. Sprinkle with salt. Do a taste test and adjust if needed.
- Pour over salad and toss to combine.
- Place into the refrigerator for at least one hour.
- Divide into four plates and top with olives.

Treats

Cinnamon Smoothie

This recipe makes 2 servings, and contains 492 calories; 47 grams fat; 18 grams protein; 6 grams net carbohydrates per serving

What You Need

- Coconut milk, 2 c
- Vanilla, .5 tsp.
- Cinnamon, 1 tsp.
- Liquid stevia, 5 drops
- Vanilla protein powder, 1 tsp.

What to Do

- Simply add everything to your blender and mix until it forms a smooth consistency
- Divide into two glasses and enjoy.

Blueberry Smoothie

This recipe makes 2 servings, and contains 353 calories; 32 grams fat; 15 grams protein; 6 grams net carbohydrates per serving

What You Need

- Spinach, 1 c
- Coconut milk, 1 c
- Mint, 4 sprigs – garnish
- Ice cubes, 4
- Coconut oil, 2 tbsp.
- Plain protein powder, 1 tsp.

- Blueberries, .5 c
- Chopped English cucumber, .5

What to Do

- Simply add everything to your blender, except for the mint, and mix until it forms a smooth consistency.
- Divide into two glasses and garnish with mint.

Vanilla Ice Cream

This recipe makes 1 serving, and contains 238 calories; 22 grams fat; 5 grams protein; 2 grams net carbohydrates per serving

What You Need

- Vanilla, 1 tbsp.
- Heavy cream, 1.25 c
- Erythritol, .5 c
- Cream of tartar, .25 tsp.
- Eggs, 4

What to Do

- Separate the eggs. Beat the cream of tartar into the egg whites. As the egg whites start to thicken up, mix in the erythritol. Continue to whisk the eggs whites until they form stiff peaks.
- Using a different bowl beat the cream. Whisk until it forms soft peaks form. Make sure that you don't overbeat the whipping cream.
- In another bowl, mix the vanilla and the egg yolks.
- Carefully fold the whipped cream and egg whites together.
- Carefully fold the egg yolk mixture into everything. You don't want to cause the mixture to fall, but you want to make sure everything is well mixed.
- Pour this into a loaf pan and freeze for at least two hours. Let it set at room temp for a few minutes to make it easier to scoop out.

Brownies

This recipe makes 16 servings, and contains 136 calories; 12 grams fat; 1 gram protein; 4 grams net carbohydrates per serving

What You Need

- Salt, .25 tsp.
- Baking powder, .5 tsp.
- Unsweetened cocoa powder, 100 g
- Powdered erythritol, 170 g
- Eggs, 3
- Almond butter, 1 c

What to Do

- Start by placing your oven to 325.
- Mix together the erythritol and almond butter using a food processor.
- Add in the salt, baking powder, cocoa powder, and eggs. Blend everything together until smooth.
- Grease a square baking dish and pour into the prepared baking dish. Bake for 12 minutes.
- Allow the brownies to cool for 30 minutes before slicing it into 16 squares. Enjoy.

Pecan Peanut Butter Bars

This recipe makes 12 servings, and contains 225 calories; 22 grams fat; 2 grams protein; 4 grams net carbohydrates per serving

What You Need

- Vanilla, 1 tsp.
- Peanut butter, .5 c

- Coconut oil, .5 c
- Pecans, 2 c

What to Do

- Grease a casserole dish and spread the pecans in the bottom of the dish.
- Add the oil and peanut butter to a microwavable bowl. Microwave it for 30 seconds. Whisk, and continue until everything has melted together.
- Add in the vanilla.
- Top the pecans with the mixture. Refrigerate this for about an hour or until set.

Peanut Butter Cookie

This recipe makes 12 servings, and contains 80 calories; 5 grams fat; 2 grams protein; 6 grams net carbohydrates per serving

What You Need

- Egg, 1
- Powdered erythritol, .5 c
- Peanut butter, 1 c

What to Do

- Start by placing the oven to 350.
- Stir everything together.
- Line a baking sheet with parchment and form 1-inch balls of dough, laying them on the baking sheet.
- Press the cookies down with a fork.
- Bake for 12 minutes.
- Allow them to cook for five minutes before serving.

Strawberry Butter

This recipe makes 48 servings, and contains 23 calories; 2 grams fat; 0 gram protein; 1 gram net carbohydrates per serving

What You Need

- Vanilla, 1 tsp.
- Lemon juice, .5 tbsp.
- Shredded unsweetened coconut, 2 c
- Strawberries, .75 c
- Coconut oil, 1 tbsp.

What You Need

- Add the coconut to your food processor and mix until it forms a paste. This is going to take around 15 minutes.
- Add in the coconut oil, strawberries, lemon juice, and vanilla into the coconut puree. Process everything together until it becomes smooth. You may want to scrape the sides of the processor down from time to time.
- Pour this through a fine mesh sieve to get rid of the strawberry seeds if you want a smooth consistency. Using the back of the spoon can help you to push everything through.
- Pour into an airtight container and then refrigerate. It will need to be kept in the refrigerator. This will last for two weeks.

Peanut Butter Mousse

This recipe makes 4 servings, and contains 280 calories; 28 grams fat; 6 grams protein; 3 grams net carbohydrates per serving

What You Need

- Heavy cream, 1 c
- Peanut butter, .25 c
- Vanilla, 1 tsp.

- Liquid stevia, 4 drops

What to Do

- Add everything to a bowl and beat together until it forms stiff peaks. This will take about five minutes. If you have a stand mixer, it will be easier on your hand.
- Spoon into four individual servings bowls and refrigerate for 30 minutes before servings.

Peanut Butter Cups

This recipe makes 6 servings, and contains 231 calories; 15 grams fat; 2 grams protein; 3 grams net carbohydrates per serving

What You Need

- Vanilla, .25 tsp.
- Stevia, .5 tsp.
- Cocoa powder, 1 tbsp.
- Unsweetened baker's chocolate, 1 oz.
- Coconut oil, .25 c
- Peanut butter, .25 c

What to Do

- Add the chocolate to a pot and let it melt. Make sure you watch the chocolate close so that it doesn't burn.
- Stir in the peanut butter. The softer your peanut butter is, the easier it will be to mix in. Mix in the coconut oil and cocoa powder next, stirring until completely mixed.
- You can use silicone molds or paper-lined cupcake tins. Pour the chocolate mixture into the cupcake molds.
- Place this in the freezer and let it set up until solid. This will take about an hour. Once they have set up, you can remove them from the molds and keep them stored in an airtight container. You can also leave them in the molds if you would like. They should be kept in the refrigerator.

Mound Bars

This recipe makes 16 servings, and contains 43 calories; 5 grams fat; 1 gram protein; 1 gram net carbohydrates per serving

What You Need

- Coconut oil, .33 c
- Shredded unsweetened coconut, .25 c
- Unsweetened cocoa powder, .25 c
- Salt
- Liquid stevia, 4 drops

What to Do

- Line a 6-inch square casserole dish with some parchment paper and set to the side.
- Add the coconut oil, salt, cocoa, and Stevie to a pot. Mix everything together until melted and combined. This will take about three minutes.
- Stir in the coconut and then press the mixture into the prepared casserole dish.
- Refrigerate the bars until they are hardened. This will take about 30 minutes.
- Once they are set, slice into 16 pieces and keep them stored in a cool place and in an airtight container.

Peppermint Mocha Drops

This recipe makes 6 servings, and contains 183 calories; 19 grams fat; 0 gram protein; 3 grams net carbohydrates per serving

What You Need

- Softened coconut oil, .25 c
- Vanilla, .5 tsp.
- Softened butter, .25 c

- Peppermint extract, 2 tsp.
- Melted dark chocolate, .33 c
- Liquid stevia, 40 drops

What to Do

- Simply place everything in a blender and combine until it forms a smooth mixture.
- Using six small silicon baking cups, scoop two tablespoons of the mixture into the cups.
- Place these molds in the freezer until they become hard. This will take about 15 minutes. Keep them stored in the refrigerator or in the freezer.
- When you are ready to use them, add a drop to a blender along with a cup of coffee and blend until smooth.

Mocha Bonbons

This recipe makes 15 servings, and contains 112 calories; 13 grams fat; 6 grams protein; 3 grams net carbohydrates per serving

What You Need

- Softened cream cheese, 8 oz.
- Coffee beans, 15 pieces
- Strong coffee, .25 c
- Cocoa butter, 2 tbsp.
- Truvia, .25 c
- MCT oil, 3 tbsp.
- Cocoa, 2 tbsp.
- Dark chocolate chips, .66 c

What to Do

- Place the softened cream cheese, cocoa, sweetener, and coffee in a stand mixer. Slowly increase the speed of the mixer; you don't want to sling the coffee everywhere.

Continue to mix until the mixture is combined and fluffy. Chill the cream cheese mixture for four hours, or overnight.

- Using a small cookie scoop, scoop out the mixture into 15 balls onto wax paper. Allow the balls to freeze for half an hour.

- Melt together the MCT oil, cocoa butter, and chocolate in the microwave. Be careful not to let the chocolate burn.

- Cover the truffles with the chocolate and press a coffee bean into the top of each truffle. Freeze for an hour and keep stored in an airtight container.

Herb Crusted Goat Cheese

This recipe makes 4 servings, and contains 304 calories; 28 grams fat; 12 grams protein; 2 grams net carbohydrates per serving

What You Need

- Chopped parsley, 1 tbsp.
- Goat cheese log, 8 oz.
- Chopped oregano, 1 tbsp.
- Pepper
- Chopped thyme, 1 tsp.
- Chopped walnuts, 6 oz.

What to Do

- Put the pepper, thyme, parsley, oregano, and walnuts into a food processor and pulse until everything is chopped fine.
- Place this mixture onto a plate. Gently roll the cheese log in the walnuts. Press slightly to adhere the walnuts onto the cheese.
- Slice and enjoy.

Coconut Chips

This recipe makes 4 servings, and contains 261 calories; 27 grams fat; 2.3 grams protein; 3 grams net carbohydrates per serving

What You Need

- Desiccated coconut, 2 cups
- Curry powder, 1 tsp.
- Salt, .5 tsp.
- Cayenne, .25 tsp.
- Garlic powder, 1 tsp.
- Melted EVOO, 2 tbsp.

What to Do

- You need to warm your oven to 350. Line a cooking sheet with parchment.
- Place the coconut, salt, spices, and coconut oil into a bowl. Stir to combine.
- Spread coconut onto the prepared baking sheet and bake for five minutes.
- Carefully take out of the oven and let cool completely.

Cashew Bars

This recipe makes 2 servings, and contains 190 calories; 18 grams fat; 4 grams protein; 2 grams net carbohydrates per serving

What You Need

- Salt
- Cinnamon, 1 tsp.
- Melted butter, .25 c
- Shredded coconut, .25 c
- Maple syrup, .25 c
- Cashews, .5 c
- Almond flour, 1 c

What to Do

- Place a sheet of parchment paper onto a baking sheet.
- Place the melted butter and almond flour into a bowl. Add in the salt, cinnamon, maple syrup, and shredded coconut. Stir well to combine.
- Chop one-half cup of the cashews and add these to the dough.
- Spread dough onto the prepared baking sheet.
- Put into the refrigerator and leave for three hours.
- Cut evenly into bars and enjoy.

Pizza Chips

This recipe makes 8 servings, and contains 250 calories; 19 grams fat; 16 grams protein; 3 grams net carbohydrates per serving

What You Need

- Italian seasoning, 2 tsp.
- Shredded Parmesan, 8 oz.
- Shredded mozzarella, 8 oz.
- Sliced pepperoni, 10 oz.

What to Do

- You need to warm your oven to 400.
- Take two baking sheets and line them with aluminum foil.
- Place the pepperoni evenly in one layer onto the prepared baking sheet.
- Sprinkle each piece with Italian seasoning, parmesan, and mozzarella.
- Put into the oven for ten minutes.
- Take out of the oven and allow to cool for five minutes or until they have turned crispy.
- If you want to, you can dip these in marinara.

Coconut Candy

This recipe makes 10 servings, and contains 104 calories; 11 grams fat; 0 gram protein; 1 gram net carbohydrates per serving

What You Need

- Sweetener, 1 tsp.
- Unsweetened shredded coconut, 1 oz.
- Melted coconut oil, .33 c
- Softened coconut butter, .33 c

What to Do

- Mix everything together until the sweetener is dissolved and everything is well combined.
- Pour into silicone molds or a cupcake tin that has been lined with paper liners. Refrigerate for one hour.
- Keep stored in the refrigerator in an airtight container.

Chocolate Mint Fat Bombs

This recipe makes 6 servings, and contains 161 calories; 19 grams fat; 0 gram protein; 1 gram net carbohydrates per serving

What You Need

- Peppermint extract, .5 tsp.
- Melted coconut oil, .5 c
- Sweetener, 1 tbsp.
- Cocoa powder, 2 tbsp.

What to Do

- Add the sweetener and peppermint extract to the melted coconut oil.

- Pour half of this mixture into another bowl along with the cocoa powder.
- Place paper liners into a cupcake tin and pour half of the chocolate mixture into the liners. Put this in the refrigerator and leave for ten minutes.
- Remove from the chocolate out of the fridge and pour in the mint mixture. Refrigerate for another ten minutes.
- Take out of the refrigerator and pour the rest of the chocolate on top. Refrigerate once again to let this layer harden.
- Unmold and enjoy.
- Keep these refrigerated.

Mini Strawberry Cheesecakes

This recipe makes 8 servings, and contains 129 calories; 13 grams fat; 2 grams protein; 2 grams net carbohydrates per serving

What You Need

- Vanilla, 1 tsp.
- Liquid stevia, 10 to 15 drops
- Softened coconut oil, .25 c
- Softened cream cheese, .75 c
- Mashed strawberries, .5 c

What to Do

- Mix everything together with a hand mixer. You could also do this with a blender.
- Take a mini muffin tin and place paper liners into each one. Carefully fill each cup with mixture.
- Place in the freezer. Let freeze for two hours.
- These should be kept in the refrigerator.

Avocado Crunch Bombs

This recipe makes 8 servings, and contains 151 calories; 14 grams fat; 3 grams protein; 5

grams net carbohydrates per serving

What You Need

- Sliced bacon, 4
- Avocados, 2
- Pecans, 6

What to Do

- Place a skillet on top of the stove on medium heat until crispy. Drain the bacon.
- Allow to cool. When cooled, crumble bacon.
- Slice the avocados in half lengthwise, open and carefully remove the pit. Spoon out the flesh and place into a bowl. Mash well. Add some lemon or lime juice to keep avocados from oxidizing.
- You can either chop the pecans with a knife or put them into a food processor and pulse until chopped.
- Place the bacon and pecans into the mashed avocados. Mix well until everything is thoroughly incorporated.
- Use a small ice cream scoop to make balls.
- Keep refrigerated.

Pumpkin Mug Cake

This recipe makes 1 serving, and contains 385 calories; 31 grams fat; 14 grams protein; 3 grams net carbohydrates per serving

What You Need

- Liquid stevia, 5 to 10 drops
- Baking soda, pinch
- Pumpkin puree, 2 tbsp.
- Pumpkin spice mix, .5 tsp.
- Erythritol, 2 tbsp.

- Egg, 1
- Ground chia seeds, 1 tbsp.
- Almond flour, 2 tbsp.
- Coconut oil, 1 tbsp.
- Coconut flour, 1 tbsp.

What to Do

- Put all the ingredients into a microwave safe mug. Stir well to combine. Microwave for two minutes on high.

Snacks and Sides

Bacon Deviled Eggs

This recipe makes 12 servings, and contains 85 calories; 7 grams fat; 6 grams protein; 2 grams net carbohydrates per serving

What You Need

- Cooked, chopped bacon, 6 slices
- Pepper
- Dijon, .5 tsp.
- Shredded Swiss cheese, .25 c
- Chopped avocado, .25
- Mayonnaise, .25 c
- Hardboiled eggs, 6

What to Do

- Slice the eggs in half lengthwise.
- Carefully take the yolks out and place them in a bowl. Lay the whites on a plate with the hollow-side up.
- Break the yolks apart with a fork and mix in the Dijon, cheese, avocado, and mayonnaise. Season with a bit of pepper.
- Spoon the yolks into the egg whites and top with some crumbled bacon. Enjoy.

Parmesan Chips

This recipe makes 4 servings, and contains 227 calories; 16 grams fat; 13 grams protein; 7 grams net carbohydrates per serving

What You Need

- Garlic powder, .5 tsp.

- Rosemary, 1 tsp.
- Almond flour, 4 tbsp.
- Grated parmesan, 6 oz.

What to Do

- Start by placing your oven to 350.
- Combine the almond flour and parmesan cheese together. Mix in the garlic powder and rosemary. Mix until everything is well combined.
- Line a baking sheet with parchment, and place tablespoon size circles of the cheese mixture.
- Bake for 10-15 minutes.
- Allow the chips to cool before servings.

Kale Chips

This recipe makes 2 servings, and contains 107 calories; 7 grams fat; 4 grams protein; 5 grams net carbohydrates per serving

What You Need

- Pepper
- Salt
- Kale leaves, 12 pieces
- Olive oil, 3 tsp.

What to Do

- Start by placing your oven to 350.
- Lay some parchment on a cooking sheet.
- Wash the kale and thoroughly dry. Lay them out on the baking sheet. Drizzle them with the oil and top with pepper and salt.
- Bake the chips for 10-15 minutes. Enjoy.

Bacon Fat Bombs

This recipe makes 12 servings, and contains 89 calories; 8 grams fat; 3 grams protein; 0 gram net carbohydrates per serving

What You Need

- Room temp cream cheese, 2 oz.
- Room temp goat cheese, 2 oz.
- Pepper
- Chopped, cooked bacon, 8 slices
- Room temp, butter, .25 c

What to Do

- Place parchment on a baking sheet and set to the side.
- Mix together the pepper, bacon, butter, cream cheese, and goat cheese in a bowl until well combined.
- Place tablespoon size mounds on the baking sheet and place in the freezer until they are firm but not completely frozen. This will take about an hour.
- These will keep in an airtight container for about two weeks.

Golden Rosti

This recipe makes 8 servings, and contains 171 calories; 15 grams fat; 5 grams protein; 3 grams net carbohydrates per serving

What You Need

- Butter, 2 tbsp.
- Minced garlic, 2 tsp.
- Chopped bacon, 8 slices
- Pepper

- Shredded acorn squash, 1 c
- Salt
- Shredded celeriac, 1 c
- Chopped thyme, 1 tsp.
- Grated parmesan, 2 tbsp.

What to Do

- Add the bacon to a large skillet and cook until crispy.
- While the bacon is cooking, mix together the squash, thyme, celeriac, garlic, and parmesan. Add in a generous amount of pepper and salt. Place this to the side.
- Drain the bacon. Once cooled, break the bacon into the rosti mixture. Mix everything together.
- Reserve two tablespoons of the bacon fat, and to the skillet along with the butter.
- Resume the heat and add in the rosti mixture and spread it around to create a large patty that is around an inch thick.
- Cook the rosti until it has browned on the bottom and crisped up.
- Flip over and then cook it on the others until it has crisped up and is cooked all the way through.
- Remove from the pan and then slice it into eight equal pieces.

Broccoli Cheddar Tots

This recipe makes 2 servings, and contains 319 calories; 22 grams fat; 21 grams protein; 7 grams net carbohydrates per serving

What You Need

- Broccoli florets, 2 c
- Cooking spray
- Eggs, 2
- Salt, 1 tsp.
- Sharp cheddar cheese, .5 c

- Almond flour, .25 c
- Parmesan, .25 c
- Coconut flour, 2 tbsp.
- Diced onion, .25 c

What to Do

- Start by placing your oven to 400. Place some parchment on a baking sheet.
- Add the broccoli to a microwavable bowl and cover it with a damp towel. Microwave the broccoli for two minutes.
- Remove the broccoli from the bowl and finely chop it. Add it back to the bowl and add in all of the remaining ingredients. Stir everything together until well combined.
- Using a tablespoon, scoop out the broccoli mixture and form them into tot shapes.
- Lay them on the baking sheet. Continue doing this until you have used all of the broccoli mixtures. Spritz the tops of the tots with the cooking spray and bake them for six minutes. Flip the tots and bake for another seven minutes.

Pecorino Mushroom Burgers

This recipe makes 4 servings, and contains 370 calories; 30 grams fat; 16 grams protein; 8 grams net carbohydrates per serving

What You Need

- Pecorino cheese, .5 c
- Whisked eggs, 2
- Mustard, 1 tsp.
- Cajun seasoning, 1 tbsp.
- Sunflower seeds, 4 tbsp.
- Hemp seeds, 4 tbsp.
- Ground flax seeds, 4 tbsp.
- Almond flour, 4 tbsp.
- Chopped Portobello mushrooms, 2 c

- Minced garlic, 2 cloves
- Softened butter, 2 tbsp.

What to Do

- Add a tablespoon of butter to a skillet and melt. Once melted, add in the garlic and mushrooms, cooking until all of the water has cooked out of the mushrooms.
- Add the Cajun seasoning, flax seeds, sunflower seeds, eggs, mustard, hemp seeds, almond flour, cooked mushrooms, onions, and pecorino in a bowl and mix together. Form the mixture into four patties.
- Add the rest of the butter to a skillet and fry up the patties for seven minutes, flip, and cook them for another six minutes. Serve warm.

Like what you're reading? Want to hear this as an audio book? Click here to get this book for FREE when you join Audible!!

https://adbl.co/2Zcx8Hq

Roasted String Beans

This recipe makes 4 servings, and contains 121 calories; 2 grams fat; 6 grams protein; 6 grams net carbohydrates per serving

What You Need

- Pepper
- Salt
- Dried thyme, .5 tsp.
- Julienned shallots, 3
- Olive oil, 3 tbsp.
- Minced garlic, 2 cloves
- Quartered tomatoes, 3
- Quartered cremini mushrooms, 1 lb.
- Halved string beans, 2 c

What to Do

- Start by placing your oven to 450.
- Mix together the pepper, salt, thyme, shallots, olive oil, garlic, tomatoes, mushrooms, and string beans. Spread the vegetables out on a baking sheet. Make sure that the veggies are in a single layer.
- Bake the vegetables for 20-25 minutes. You can flip the veggies over halfway through the cooking process if you would like to. Enjoy.

Fries and Aioli

This recipe makes 4 servings, and contains 205 calories; 4 grams fat; 2 grams protein; 4 grams net carbohydrates per serving

What You Need

Aioli

- Lemon juice, 3 tbsp.
- Pepper
- Salt
- Minced garlic, 2 cloves
- Mayonnaise, 4 tbsp.

Fries

- Pepper
- Salt
- Chopped parsley, 5 tbsp.
- Olive oil, 2 tbsp.
- Julienned carrots, 3
- Julienned parsnips, 6

What to Do

- Start by placing your oven to 400.
- Whisk together all of the aioli ingredients together and allow the mixture to refrigerate for at least 30 minutes.
- Lay the carrots and parsnips out on a cooking sheet and drizzle them with oil. Sprinkle on the pepper and salt. Move the veggies around in the baking sheet to make sure that they are all evenly coated.
- Bake them for 35 minutes.
- Transfer the fries to a plate and garnish with the parsley. Serve them with aioli.

Garlic Mashed Celeriac

This recipe makes 4 servings, and contains 94 calories; 0 gram fat; 2 grams protein; 6 grams net carbohydrates per serving

What You Need

- Pepper
- Salt
- Dried basil, 2 tsp.
- Garlic powder, .5 tsp.
- Sour cream, .33 c
- Butter, 2 tbsp.
- Cream cheese, 2 oz.
- Water, 4 c
- Chopped celeriac, 2 lb.

What to Do

- Add the celeriac to a pot of water and boil. Let this cook for 5 minutes and then turn the heat down and let the celeriac simmer for about 15 minutes. Drain out the water.
- Put the cooked celeriac in a bowl with the pepper, salt, basil, garlic powder, sour cream, butter, and cream cheese. Use an electric mixer on medium speed to mix everything together and to create a creamy consistency. This is perfect served with grilled salmon.

Spicy Deviled Eggs

This recipe makes 12 servings, and contains 112 calories; 9 grams fat; 6 grams protein; 0 gram net carbohydrates per serving

What You Need

- Ice water bath
- Chopped parsley – garnish
- Pinch of paprika
- Dijon, .25 tsp.

- Worcestershire sauce, .5 tsp.
- Mixed dried herbs, 1 tsp.
- Chili pepper
- Salt
- Mayonnaise, 6 tbsp.
- Water, 1.5 c
- Eggs, 12

What to Do

- Bring a pot of water to a boil. Slowly and carefully ease the eggs into the boiling water. Allow them to cook for 12 minutes.
- Once the eggs have cooked drain off the hot water and place the eggs directly in an ice water bath to cool off.
- Once you can handle the eggs, peel them.
- Slice the eggs lengthwise and carefully pop the yolks out and place them in a bowl. Set the whites on a plate with the hollow side up.
- Break the yolks up with a fork. Add in the paprika, mustard, Worcestershire sauce, dried herbs, chili pepper, salt, and mayonnaise. Mix everything together until it forms a smooth paste.
- Spoon the mixture into the egg whites. If you want to make them look pretty, you can also add the yolk mixture to a piping bag and pip in rosettes.
- Garnish the top of the deviled eggs with parsley and enjoy.

Avocado Crostini

This recipe makes 4 servings, and contains 195 calories; 12 grams fat; 13 grams protein; 3 grams net carbohydrates per serving

What You Need

- Chia seeds, 1 tbsp.
- Lemon juice, 1 tsp.
- Chopped raw walnuts, .33 c

- Coconut oil, 1.5 tbsp.
- Salt, .33 tsp.
- Mashed avocado, 1 c
- Nori sheets, 4
- Low-carb baguette, 8 slices

What to Do

- Flake the nori sheets apart into small pieces and place in a bowl.
- In a separate bowl, mix together the lemon juice, salt, and avocado. Mix in the nori flakes and set to the side.
- Lay the baguette slices out on a baking sheet and toast them under the broiler for about two minutes. Make sure the bread doesn't burn.
- Take them out of the oven and brush the coconut oil on both sides of the baguette slices.
- Top the crostini with the avocado mixture and top with the walnuts and chia seeds. Enjoy.

Low-Carb Cheddar Bay Biscuits

This recipe makes 6-8 servings, and contains 153 calories; 14 grams fat; 5 grams protein; 1 gram net carbohydrates per serving

What You Need

- Greek yogurt, .33 c
- Grated sharp cheddar cheese, 1.25 c
- Melted butter, .33 c
- Eggs, 5
- Baking powder, 1 tsp.
- Salt
- Garlic powder, 2 tsp.
- Almond flour, .33 c

What to Do

- Start by placing your oven to 350.

- Mix together the cheddar cheese, baking powder, salt, garlic powder, and almond flour.

- Mix the yogurt, butter, and eggs together in another bowl. Add the yogurt mixture into the almond flour mixture. Stir everything together until it forms a biscuit-like consistency.

- Drop biscuits sized dollops of the biscuit dough onto a baking sheet. Make sure that you keep them about two inches apart.

- Bake the biscuits for 12 minutes, or until they are golden brown on top. Enjoy.

Spinach and Cheese Balls

This recipe makes 8 servings, and contains 160 calories; 15 grams fat; 8 grams protein; 1 gram net carbohydrates per serving

What You Need

- Almond flour, 1 c
- Spinach, 8 oz.
- Eggs, 2
- Garlic powder, 1 tsp.
- Parmesan, .33 c
- Melted butter, 2 tbsp.
- Onion powder, 1 tbsp.
- Heavy cream, 3 tbsp.
- Pepper, .25 tsp.
- Nutmeg, .25 tsp.
- Ricotta cheese, .33 c

What to Do

- Simply add the ingredients to a blender. Mix everything together until it forms a smooth mixture.

- Pour the mixture into a bowl and freeze for about ten minutes to firm it up slightly.

- Set your oven to 350.

- Once firm, form the mixture into balls and lay them out on a parchment-lined baking sheet.

- Bake the cheese balls for 10-12 minutes. Once browned, enjoy or store in an airtight container once cooled and keep refrigerated.

Stuffed Piquillo Peppers

This recipe makes 8 servings, and contains 132 calories; 11 grams fat; 6 grams protein; 3 grams net carbohydrates per serving

What You Need

- Balsamic vinegar, 1 tbsp.
- Prosciutto, 4 slices – sliced in half
- Olive oil, 1 tbsp.
- Roasted piquillo peppers, 8

Filling

- Chopped mint, 1 tbsp.
- Minced garlic, .5 tsp.
- Chopped parsley, 3 tbsp.
- Olive oil, 1 tbsp.
- Heavy cream, 3 tbsp.
- Goat cheese, 8 oz.

What to Do

- Mix the filling ingredients together. Add the filling to a freezer bag and push the mixture to the corner of the bag. Trim off the corner.

- Take the peppers and clean out the inside. Add about two tablespoons of the filling mixture into each of the peppers.
- Wrap a slice of prosciutto around each of the peppers. Secure the prosciutto with toothpicks.
- Place them on a plate and top with a drizzle of balsamic vinegar and olive oil.

Coconut Ginger Macaroons

This recipe makes 6 servings, and contains 97 calories; 3 grams fat; 6 grams protein; 0 gram net carbohydrates per serving

What You Need

- Water, 1 c
- Pinch of chili powder
- Swerve, .25 c
- Finely shredded coconut, 1 c
- Egg whites, 6
- Pureed ginger root, 2 fingers

What to Do

- Start by place the oven to 350.
- Lay some parchment on a cooking sheet.
- In a heat-safe bowl, mix together the chili powder, swerve, shredded coconut, egg whites, and ginger.
- Boil a pot of water. Make sure that the bowl with the coconut mixture can fit over the pot of water with the bottom touching the water.
- Set the bowl over the boiling water and continue to whisk the mixture until it becomes glossy. This will take about four minutes.
- Place the mixture in a piping bag fitted and pipe out around 40-50 macaroons onto your prepared baking sheet. Cook these for about 15 minutes or until browned.
- Once the macaroons are cooked, place them on a wire rack to cool. You can garnish them with some angel hair chili if you want.

Chicken Fritters with Dip

This recipe makes 4 servings, and contains 151 calories; 7 grams fat; 12 grams protein; 1 gram net carbohydrates per serving

What You Need

- Finely chopped onion, 2 tbsp.
- Garlic powder, 1 tsp.
- Chopped dill, 4 tbsp. – divided
- Chopped parsley, 1 tbsp.
- Mayonnaise, 1.25 c – divided
- Olive oil, 3 tbsp.
- Grated mozzarella, 1 c
- Pepper
- Salt
- Sour cream, 1 c
- Eggs, 2
- Coconut flour, .25 c
- Thinly sliced and chopped chicken breasts, 1 lb.

What to Do

- Mix together a cup of mayonnaise, the garlic powder, sour cream, salt, onion, parsley, and three tablespoons of dill. Cover this with saran wrap and refrigerate as you fix everything else.

- Next, mix together the rest of the dill and mayonnaise, along with the mozzarella, pepper, salt, eggs, and coconut flour. Mix in the chicken, making sure that everything is well combined. Cover up of the bowl and let the chicken marinate for at least two hours.

- Add some olive oil to a pan and heat it up. Scoop out two tablespoons of the batter and place them in the heated pan. Use your spatula to flatten the mixture out into a fritter shape.

- Let the mixture cook for four minutes on one side. Make sure the first side is very well browned and golden so that it holds together when you flip it.

- Flip the fritter, cooking for another four minutes, or until completely cooked. Set the fritter onto a wire race and continue with the rest of the batter. Add extra oil as you need to.

- Garnish the fritters with some parsley and serve with the dill dip you made earlier.

Amaretti Biscuits

This recipe makes 6 servings, and contains 165 calories; 13 grams fat; 9 grams protein; 3 grams net carbohydrates per serving

What You Need

- Powdered swerve, .75 c – topping
- Softened butter, .25 c
- Mascarpone cheese, .25 c
- Amaretto whiskey, 7 tbsp.
- Juice of a lemon
- Ground almonds, .25 c
- Pinch of salt
- Powdered swerve, 8 oz.
- Vanilla bean paste, 1 tsp.
- Beaten egg yolk
- Egg whites, 6

What to Do

- Start by placing your oven on 300 and place some parchment paper on a baking sheet.
- Beat together the vanilla paste, salt, and egg whites using an electric mixer. As you are mixing the egg whites, slowly add in the 8 ounces of the powdered Swerve. Keep mixing until the egg whites form stiff peaks.
- Mix together the amaretto, lemon juice, egg yolk, and ground almonds. Carefully fold this mixture into the egg whites.

- Add the batter to a piping bag and form 40-50 mounds onto your prepared baking sheet. Bake the biscuits for 15 minutes. They should be golden brown.

- Whisk together the remaining swerve, butter, and mascarpone cheese. Set to the side.

- Once the biscuits are cooked through. Remove to a wire rack and allow them to cool. Place some of the mascarpone cheese mixtures onto half of the biscuits, on the flat side. Press another biscuit onto each, forming a sandwich. Sift on some extra powdered swerve if desired.

Pesto Parmesan Dip

This recipe makes 6 servings, and contains 161 calories; 14 grams fat; 5 grams protein; 3 grams net carbohydrates per serving

What You Need

- Pepper
- Salt
- Sliced olives, 8
- Grated parmesan cheese, .5 c
- Pesto, 2 tbsp.
- Cream cheese, 1 c

What to Do

- Mix all of the ingredients together
- Place into the refrigerator for 20 minutes.
- Keep refrigerated.

Bacon Dip

This recipe makes 12 servings, and contains 190 calories; 17 grams fat; 7 grams protein; 4 grams net carbohydrates per serving

What You Need

- Sliced scallions, 1 c
- Shredded cheddar, 1 c
- Cream cheese, 1 c
- Sour cream, 1.5 c
- Sliced bacon, 5

What to Do

- You need to warm your oven to 400.
- Cook the bacon until crispy. Drain the cooked bacon. Once cooled, crumble.
- Place bacon along with all the other ingredients into a mixing bowl. Combine everything together.
- Pour into a baking dish.
- Bake for 30 minutes.
- Allow to cool for ten minutes before serving.

Cheddar Chips

This recipe makes 4 servings, and contains 457 calories; 38 grams fat; 28 grams protein; 1 gram net carbohydrates per serving

What You Need

- Shredded cheddar, 4 c
- Salt

What to Do

- You need to warm your oven to 350.
- Lay a sheet of parchment paper on a cooking sheet.
- Spoon the cheese into mounds onto the prepared baking sheet.
- Place in oven for five minutes. Check frequently until cheese is browned. Don't let it burn.

- Sprinkle the cheese with salt.
- Allow to cool completely.

Nachos

This recipe makes 2 to 4 servings, and contains 599 calories; 45 grams fat; 41 grams protein; 5 grams net carbohydrates per serving

What You Need

- Shredded cheddar, 2 c
- Pork rinds, 1.5 oz. bag
- Pepper
- Chopped cilantro, 1 tbsp.
- Salt
- Lime juice, 1.5 tsp.
- Minced jalapeno, 1
- Minced garlic, 1 tsp.
- Chopped onion, .25
- Chopped tomato, 1 medium

What to Do

- Place the tomato, onion, cilantro, jalapeno, garlic, and lime juice into a bowl. Sprinkle with pepper and salt. Stir well to combine. Set to the side for one hour.
- You need to warm your oven to 350. Place aluminum foil onto a rimmed baking sheet.
- Place the pork rinds in one layer onto the prepared baking sheet. Sprinkle to cheese on top and then spoon on the salsa.
- Place into the oven for 15 minutes. Remove carefully. Place onto a serving platter and enjoy.

Queso

This recipe makes 6 servings, and contains 213 calories; 19 grams fat; 10 grams protein; 2 grams net carbohydrates per serving

What You Need

- Cayenne pepper, .25 tsp.
- Shredded cheddar, 6 oz.
- Goat cheese, 2 oz.
- Onion powder, .5 tsp.
- Minced garlic, 1 tsp.
- Diced, seeded, jalapeno, .5
- Coconut milk, .5 cup

What to Do

- Place the onion powder, garlic, jalapeno, and coconut milk into a saucepan. Stir to combine.
- Bring everything to a simmer. Add in goat cheese and whisk until completely smooth.
- Place the cayenne and cheddar into the pan and continue to whisk until thickened.
- Serve with vegetables or keto-friendly crackers.

Parmesan Crackers

This recipe makes 8 servings, and contains 133 calories; 11 grams fat; 11 grams protein; 1 gram net carbohydrates per serving

What You Need

- Grated Parmesan cheese, 8 oz.
- Butter, 1 tsp.

What to Do

- You need to warm your oven to 450.
- Line a cooking sheet with parchment. Grease with one teaspoon of butter.
- Put the Parmesan cheese on the baking sheet in mounds placed evenly apart.
- Bake until edges have browned around five minutes.
- Take out of the oven and gently use a spatula to place them on paper towels. Blot any excess grease from the tops with paper towels. Let them completely cool.

Asparagus and Walnuts

This recipe makes 4 servings, and contains 124 calories; 12 grams fat; 3 grams protein; 2 grams net carbohydrates per serving

What You Need

- Chopped walnuts, .25 c
- Pepper
- Salt
- Trimmed asparagus, .75 lb.
- Olive oil, 1.5 tbsp.

What to Do

- Place a large skillet on top of the stove and warm the olive oil on medium heat.
- Cook the asparagus until tender and slightly browned. This will take about five minutes.
- Sprinkle with pepper and salt.
- Take out of the skillet and add the walnuts. Toss to combine.

Garlicky Green Beans

This recipe makes 4 servings, and contains 104 calories; 9 grams fat; 4 grams protein; 1 gram net carbohydrates per serving

What You Need

- Grated Parmesan, .25 c
- Olive oil, 2 tbsp.
- Pepper
- Salt
- Minced garlic, 1 tsp.
- Steamed green beans, 1 lb.

What to Do

- You need to warm your oven to 425.
- Lay some parchment on a cooking sheet.
- Sprinkle with pepper and salt.
- Spread evenly onto baking sheet. Place into the oven for ten minutes. Beans should be tender and slightly browned.
- Sprinkle on Parmesan cheese and enjoy.

Creamed Spinach

This recipe makes 4 servings, and contains 195 calories; 20 grams fat; 3 grams protein; 1 gram net carbohydrates per serving

What You Need

- Pepper
- Salt
- Nutmeg
- Chicken broth, .25 c
- Heavy cream, .75 c
- Spinach, 4 c

- Thinly sliced small onion
- Butter, 1 tbsp.

What to Do

- Place a skillet on top of the stove and melt the butter on medium heat.
- Cook the onions until slightly caramelized around five minutes.
- Put the nutmeg, pepper, salt, chicken broth, heavy cream, and spinach into the skillet. Stir well to combine.
- Cook until spinach is tender and sauce is thick. This will take about 15 minutes.

Zucchini Crisps

This recipe makes 4 servings, and contains 94 calories; 8 grams fat; 4 grams protein; 1 gram net carbohydrates per serving

What You Need

- Pepper
- Grated Parmesan cheese, .5 c
- Sliced zucchini, 4
- Butter, 2 tbsp.

What to Do

- Slice the zucchini into round slices that are about a fourth-inch circle.
- Place a large skillet on top of the stove and melt the butter on medium.
- Cook the zucchini in the pan, cooking until tender and browned.
- Sprinkle with Parmesan.
- Cook until cheese is melted and crispy. This will take an additional five minutes.

Mashed Cheesy Cauliflower

This recipe makes 4 servings, and contains 183 calories; 15 grams fat; 8 grams protein; 4 grams net carbohydrates per serving

What You Need

- Pepper
- Salt
- Room temp butter, 2 tbsp.
- Heavy cream, .25 c
- Shredded cheddar, .5 c
- Chopped cauliflower, 1 head

What to Do

- Place the chopped cauliflower into a saucepan and put water into it that covers the cauliflower.
- Place on top of the stove and let it come to a boil.
- Let this boil for five minutes and pour into a colander. Let it drain completely.
- Place into a food processor and break up into smaller pieces. Add in butter, cream, and cheese. Process until whipped and creamy.
- Add pepper and salt to taste.

Mushroom and Camembert

This recipe makes 4 servings, and contains 161 calories; 13 grams fat; 9 grams protein; 3 grams net carbohydrates per serving

What You Need

- Pepper
- Diced Camembert, 4 oz.
- Halved button mushrooms, 1 lb.

- Minced garlic, 2 tsp.
- Butter, 2 tbsp.

What to Do

- Place a skillet on top of the stove and melt the butter on medium heat.
- Place the garlic in the skillet and cook until fragrant.
- Add mushrooms continue to cook until tender around ten minutes.
- Add in cheese and cook until melted.
- Add pepper, taste and adjust seasonings if needed.

Zucchini Noodles with Pesto

This recipe makes 4 servings, and contains 93 calories; 8 grams fat; 4 grams protein; 2 grams net carbohydrates per serving

What You Need

- Grated Parmesan cheese, .25 c
- Zucchini, 4
- EVOO, .25 c
- Nutritional yeast, 2 tsp.
- Garlic cloves, 3
- Basil leaves, 1 c
- Chopped kale, 1 c

What to Do

- Place the yeast, garlic, basil, and kale into a food processor. Process until finely chopped.
- Keeping the food processor on low, drizzle in the olive oil until it forms a thick paste. Add some water if it gets too thick.

- Either use a peeler to turn the zucchini into "noodles" or use a spiralizer. Place into a bowl.
- Stir in pesto and parmesan cheese. Give everything a good toss to get everything coated.

Bacon and Blue Cheese Zoodles

This recipe makes 1 serving, and contains 435 calories; 33 grams fat; 21 grams protein; 5 grams net carbohydrates per serving

What You Need

- Pepper
- Cooked and crumbled bacon, .5 c
- Crumbled blue cheese, .33 c
- Blue cheese dressing, 3 tbsp.
- Baby spinach, .5 cup
- Spiralized zucchini, 1 c

What to Do

- Put all ingredients into a bowl. Toss well to coat. Serve.
- If you don't have a spiralizer, you can get the same effect by using a peeler.

Conclusion

Thank for making it through to the end of *30-Day Ketogenic Meal Plan*, let's hope it was informative and able to provide you with all of the tools you need to achieve your goals whatever they may be.

A ketogenic diet is a great way to lose weight and get healthy. With planning and tons of recipes at your disposal, you are sure to be successful. The key to seeing results is to make the diet as easy as possible. Creating a meal plan can do just that. Use the information you have learned in this book to do just that.

Diets don't have to be boring. In fact, the more fun and variety you can have with a diet, the easier it will be. The limitless number of meal plan creations you can make with the recipes found in this book is sure to keep you interested. Don't continue to put off changing the way you eat. Make the change today, and you will see the results.

Finally, if you found this book useful in any way, a review on Amazon is always appreciated!

Description

Have you been considering a ketogenic diet? Are you unsure where to start and how hard it's going to be? If you answered yes, then this book is for you.

A ketogenic diet is a great way to lose weight and get healthy. The great news is, it doesn't have to be difficult, hard, or confusing. With enough recipes and a basic understanding of macros, you can be successful. This book is here to help you do just that.

In this book you will find:

- Basic information on the keto diet
- How to create a meal plan
- A 30-day meal plan
- Lots of recipes
- And much more

Some of the tasty recipes you will find in here include:

- Creamy Butter Chicken
- Taco Salad
- Cinnamon Smoothie
- Sausage Crust Pizza
- Thai Lettuce Wraps
- Coconut Ginger Macaroons

Meal plans are a great way to make sure that you stick to a diet. Once you have a good list of recipes, and you know what your macros are, you can easily create your own meal plan. With the help of this book, you will get a feel of what a meal plan should look like, which will make your life easier when it comes to creating your own.

Don't wait any longer. Get this book today and learn how to lead a healthy life with the ketogenic diet.

www.ingramcontent.com/pod-product-compliance
Lightning Source LLC
Chambersburg PA
CBHW081154020426
42333CB00020B/2495